THE CLINICAL APPLICATION OF MMPI SPECIAL SCALES

Eugene E. Levitt, Ph. D.

Indiana University School of Medicine

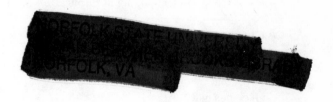

 LAWRENCE ERLBAUM ASSOCIATES, PUBLISHERS
1989 Hillsdale, New Jersey   Hove and London

Lawrence Erlbaum Associates, Inc., Publishers
365 Broadway
Hillsdale, New Jersey 07642

Library of Congress Cateloging in Publication Data

Levitt, Eugene E.
    The clinical application of MMPI special scales / Eugene E.
Levitt.
        p. cm.
    Includes index.
    ISBN 0-8058-0047-6
    1. Minnesota Multiphasic Personality Inventory. 2. Mental
illness--Diagnosis. 3. Adjustment (Psychology)--Testing.
    I. Title.
    RC473.M5L48 1989   88-21272
    616.89'075--dc19   CIP

PRINTED IN THE UNITED STATES OF AMERICA
10 9 8 7 6 5 4 3 2 1

This book is dedicated with affection,
admiration, respect and gratitude to a man whom
I have with great pride called friend,
colleague and leader for more than three decades

John Ignatius Nurnberger, M.D.

Distinguished Professor Emeritus of Psychiatry
Indiana University School of Medicine

Contents

Chapter 1 - Introduction

Chapter 2 - The Validity Measures

Chapter 3 - Some Useful Special Scales

Chapter 4 - The Assessment of Psychopathology

Chapter 5 - The Measurement of Adjustment and Personality

Chapter 6 - MMPI Special Scales and the Rorschach

Appendixes

Foreword

The Minnesota Multiphasic Personality Inventory was designed to provide, in a single diagnostic instrument, a comprehensive assessment of a number of psychiatric syndromes and personality characteristics manifested by persons with various types of psychological disorders. Consistent with this goal, the MMPI clinical scales were intended to identify individuals with specific behavioral disorders. However, research has shown that the clinical scales are not fully adequate to these tasks. Consequently, MMPI interpretation of abnormal personality traits is now based primarily on high point codes and profile patterns, rather than on individual clinical scales.

Limitations in the descriptive power of the original MMPI clinical scales has stimulated the development of a large number of special scales. Psychologists who work with the MMPI have creatively devised supplementary or special scales from the rich pool of 550 MMPI items describing diverse psychological and medical symptoms. These special scales provide relevant and specific assessment information about a wide range of psychodiagnostic and treatment problems that cannot be adequately assessed with the MMPI clinical scales.

More than a decade ago, Dahlstrom, Welsh, and Dahlstrom (1972 , 1975) reported the existence of more than 450 special scales. By now there are undoubtedly more special scales than MMPI items, as Butcher and Tellegen (1978) more recently noted. Unfortunately, the titles given to special scales are often misleading, relatively little reliability and validity information is available for many of these scales, and cross validation efforts are generally inadequate or totally lacking. Typically, special scales have been neglected and largely ignored. Professor Levitt's is the first book to deal entirely with special scales as diagnostic tools. High point codes and clinical profiles have no role in Levitt's approach to psychodiagnosis with the MMPI .

This unique volume fulfills the need for a comprehensive, authoritative review and critical evaluation of many MMPI special scales. Levitt shares with us the wisdom and insight he has gleaned from reviewing more than 150 special scales in thousands of MMPI records obtained from diverse psychiatric and medical inpatient and outpatient samples and a variety of normal populations. Vital information and guidelines are provided for interpreting the most useful MMPI special scales, including some the author has found especially effective in his own clinical practice that are practically unknown, and several scales that have never before been published. The MMPI special scales featured herein have stood the critical test of time in terms of their clinical utility.

Based on three decades of clinical experience at the Indiana University Medical Center, Levitt's provocative thesis is that MMPI special scales provide more accurate and useful information for the clinical practitioner than the traditional MMPI scales. The practicing clinician is given detailed guidance on how to interpret more than 55 special scales—information that can be immediately applied in reviewing patients' MMPI records. The contents should prove invaluable for practicing clinicians, researchers and students of the MMPI.

Potentially fruitful and needed research with these scales is also noted.

The statistical statements concerning the special scales that are reported in this book are based on comparisons of individuals and groups of patients with a heterogeneous normative sample of adult subjects. Normative data were collected by Levitt and his associates on 100 normal subjects, most of them residing in the nearby community. Although Levitt's normative sample is admittedly not representative, and considerable smaller than the original MMPI normative groups, the Indiana subjects were tested subsequent to 1980 with the entire set of 550 MMPI items, in contrast to the original MMPI normative norms, which was compiled more than 40 years ago with the original set of only 504 items.

Since the revised MMPI will be published shortly, or perhaps simultaneously with this volume, one might question the timeliness of a book on the MMPI special scales. A number of the original MMPI items will be replaced, including items that are found in the currently existing special scales. However, since the clinical scales will apparently remain essentially intact, the Harris and Lingoes subscales can continue to be used in their present form. Guidelines for the interpretation of these scales provided in this volume are more comprehensive than can be found elsewhere. Moreover, it seems likely that a substantial period of transition will be required for the acceptance of the revised MMPI. Availability of accurate information about the special scales will facilitate their use during this transition period and assist in the adaptation of those special scales with proven utility in the revised MMPI. Detailed information about special scales will also facilitate research on those problems that initially stimulated the construction of the various special scales.

Over the years, the MMPI has proved to be, by a wide margin, the most useful and widely used general-purpose personality measure in both research and clinical practice. The imminent publication of the revised form can only serve to further increase the utility of this instrument. It will, no doubt, also serve to stimulate the development of new special scales. This volume provides a valuable presentation of present knowledge about MMPI special scales, a solid foundation on which more sophisticated and clinically useful special scales can be based in the future.

Charles D. Spielberger
Tampa, Florida

Acknowledgments

Even the author of a small book—if it's worth much—needs a lot of help. Despite its diminutiveness, this small book was a number of years in the making and it becomes a brain-cracking task to recall every person who contributed to my modest final product. My colleagues and interns in the Section of Psychology of the Department of Psychiatry at the Indiana University School of Medicine rank foremost among the contributors, led by James M. Brooks, Frank J. Connolly, Clayton E. Ladd, Richard J. Lawlor, Wm. George McAdoo, Nuran B. Miller, and Charles W. Perkins. Psychiatrists, social workers, other physicians, clergy, administrators, and trainees of most of these disciplines provided valuable feedback on MMPI records that is a crucial fundament of clinical lore. George H. Ritz, Jr. first showed me how to use the Harris and Lingoes subscales of the MMPI many years ago. The text benefitted substantially from a critical reading of the manuscript by Robert P. Archer.

Much solid technical assistance was the contribution of Sandra Barton, Phyllis Bramer, Helen Kronman, and Tod S. Levitt. Important statistical arrangements were the portion donated by Gregory Orr.

Many typists worked on the manuscript over the years. I can remember Vicki Wilson, Becky Agee, Cassandra Summerlot, Janet Shennib, Jane Troxell, and Jeanne Wilson. The final manuscript was the work of Lowana Alfonzo.

To all these wonderful people I acknowledge my indebtedness with gratitude and humility.

I have benefited by the experience, wisdom, and clinical skills of many colleagues of different disciplines. I take sole responsibility, however, for any evaluative statements in this book that are not directly attributable to another source, including those that are specifically acknowledged to be based on clinical use.

Eugene E. Levitt

Special Scales Key

Harris & Lingoes Scales

2SD = Subjective Depression
2PR = PsychomotorRetardation
2PM = PhysicalMalfunctioning
2MD = Mental Dullness
2B = Brooding
3DSA = Denial of Social Anxiety
3NA = Need forAffection
3LM = Lassitude and Malaise
3SC = Somatic Symptoms
3IA = Inhibition of Aggression
4FD = Familial Discord
4AC = Authority Conflict
4SI = Social Imperturbability
4SOA = Social Alienation
4SEA = Self-Alienation
6PI = Persecutory Ideas
6P = Poignancy
6N = Naivete
8SOA = Social Alienation
8EA = Emotional Alienation
8COG = Lack Of Ego Mastery, Cognitive
8CON = Lack Of Ego Mastery, Conative
8BSE = Bizarre Sensory Experiences
8DIC = Lack Of Ego Mastery, Defect of Inhibition and Control
9AMO = Amorality
9PMA = Psychomotor Acceleration
9EI = Ego Inflation
9IMP = Imperturbability

Wiggins Scales

AUT = Authority Conflict
DEP = Depression
FAM = Family Problems
FEM = Feminine Interests
HEA = Poor Health
HYP = Hypomania
HOS = Manifest Hostility
MOR = Poor Morale
ORG = Organic Symptoms
PHO = Phobias
PSY = Psychoticism
REL = Religious Fundamentalism
SOC = Social Maladjustment

Tryon, Stein, & Chu Scales

TSC/A = Autism
TSC/B = Body Symptoms
TSC/D = Depression
TSC/I = Social Introversion
TSC/R = Resentment
TSC/S = Suspicion
TSC/T = Tension

Indiana Scales

I-De = Dependency
I-Do = Dominance
I-DS = Dissociative Symptoms
I-OC = Obsessive-Compulsiveness
I-RD = Severe Reality Distortion
I-SC = Self-Concept
I-SP = Sex Problems

Other Scales

AMac = MacAndrew Alcoholism Scale
Astvn = Assertiveness
Cl = Carelessness
Cn = Control
D-S = Depression, Subtle
E/Cy = Cynicism
Ho = Hostility
ME = Mean Elevation on eight clinical scales
OH = Overcontrolled Hostility
S+ = Extreme Suspiciousness
TR = Test-Retest
WA = Work Attitude
5C = Conventionality

CHAPTER 1
INTRODUCTION

Many verbal inventories for the measurement of psychopathology and personality have been developed over the past 40 years. Some attained modest prominence at least for a time; others were neglected from the beginning and little is known about their attributes and capacities. Only a handful have survived perennially. The outstanding example is the Minnesota Multiphasic Personality Inventory (MMPI). The MMPI was born over 40 years ago but remains the most popular formal assessment tool in psychology and education. It has the deepest potential for evaluating human personality, for measuring change in personal and emotional status, for increasing the accuracy of diagnosis, and for giving useful information regarding treatment plans and prognosis. Thousands of publications, perennial workshops, and computerized interpretive programs testify to the popularity of the MMPI. An estimated 15 million MMPIs are administered in the United States alone each year.

Despite its longevity, the MMPI has a number of methodological defects that have been summarized by Faschingbauer (1979) and Levitt and Duckworth (1984). Wiener and Harmon (1946) observed early that there are two types of statements in the MMPI clinical scales: obvious and subtle. An obvious item is one for which the psychopathological or diagnostic response is clear as, for example, responding "true" to the statement "Life is a strain for me much of the time." A subtle item is one for which there is no response that is keyed for psychopathology as, for example, "I liked *Alice in Wonderland* by Lewis Carroll."

Every relevant investigation has shown that the correlations between the obvious and subtle subsections of the clinical scales range from zero to low negative, a certain mathematical argument for dimensional independence. Summing these unrelated subsets into a single score can only be a "cancellation approach" to scale scores (Norman, 1972; Faschingbauer, 1979).

The obvious–subtle differential is not the only criticism that has been leveled at MMPI clinical scales. Faschingbauer (1979) described them as "heterogeneous, redundant, and overlapping..over 100 items are not even scored. How much potentially useful information never enters the code type as a result is still unknown" (p.374). Faschingbauer is in essential agreement with Norman (1972) who pointed out that the clinical scales are not only "inefficient, redundant, and largely irrelevant for their present purposes" (p.64) but also the MMPI methods of "combining scale scores and for profile interpretation are unconscionably cumbersome and obtuse" (p.64). Norman summed up by noting that "it is abundantly clear that they are about as inappropriate and maladapted a set as one could imagine for their current uses in profile analysis, and interpretation and typal class definition" (p.64).

Wiggins (1966), commenting on the heterogeneity of the clinical scales, remarked that "the hodgepodge of content which contributes to a high score on a given clinical scale is not suggestive of any consistent personality trait or structure" (p.31). Indeed, the libraries of interpretive statements that have been proposed for high scores on clinical scales are at best unenlightening and at worst, confusing. For example, Graham (1987) listed 44 interpretive statements that can accompany a high score on Scale 4 plus 16 statements that follow from low scores. A high score on Scale 9 yields 42 interpretive statements, a low score, 14 more. Clopton (1979a) pointed out the obvious: Respondents endorsing very different subsets of items can obtain the same raw score on any scale.

Thus, to select the appropriate interpretative statements from among Graham's lists requires that the clinician examine the protocol's individual item responses. It is unsafe to make interpretations based solely on the clinical scale score.

To exemplify this phenomenon, Wiggins (1966) created profiles for two hypothetical patients whose clinical scale profiles (see Figure 1.1) were identical but whose scores on Wiggins' content scales varied markedly as indicated in Table 1.1.

Obviously, the interpretations of the two identical clinical profiles using high point codes or any other method of analysis would also be identical. Wiggins discussed the differences in interpretation of the two records according to Table 1.1.

Patient A has admitted to a larger number of symptoms thought to be indicative of organic pathology. Additionally, he admits having family problems and a number of psychotic symptoms of a primarily paranoid nature. He is greatly concerned about his health and admits to liking an unusual number of feminine pursuits. By comparison with Patient A, Patient B is generally more deviant with respect to content categories reflecting poor morale, mood instability, social maladjustment and hostility.

The configuration of content scale scores of Patient B readily confirms the impression of psychopathology gained from an inspection of the clinical profile

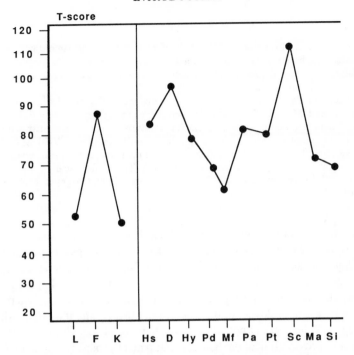

Figure 1.1 Clinical Profile of Wiggins' Hypothetical Patients

Table 1.1

**Raw Scores on Wiggins Scales for Two
Hypothetical Patients with Identical Clinical Scale Profiles**

Content scale	Patient A	Patient B	Difference
ORG	28	5	+23
PSY	8	21	-13
HEA	7	20	-13
FEM	6	17	-11
FAM	11	6	+5
DEP	15	19	-4
HYP	8	12	-4
PHO	13	9	+4
SOC	10	13	-3
HOS	9	12	-3
AUT	13	11	+2
REL	7	9	-2
MOR	12	11	+1

in Figure 1.1. This could be the profile of a paranoid schizophrenic with an underlying homosexual component and a body concern that is delusional in nature. Poor morale, social maladjustment, and hostility are, of course, compatible with this picture.

Although Patient A's raw content scale scores are sufficiently deviant to be considered those of a hospitalized patient, they are in sharp contrast to those of Patient B. By comparison, Patient A is almost exclusively concerned with organic symptoms and, to a lesser extent, family problems. Evidence of delusional thinking, health concern, feminine interests, and general maladjustment is comparatively weak for Patient A. The clinical scale profile in Figure 1.1 may now be viewed in a quite different light. (Wiggins, 1966, p. 30)

The MMPI clinical scales are not without their defenders. The thrust of the defense is that the clinical scales were intended to measure psychopathology, not personality traits and it is unfair to criticize the MMPI for being unable to do what it has never been intended to do (Dahlstrom, 1969; Butcher & Tellegen, 1978).

Thus, Dahlstrom (1969) pointed out that internal item consistency and homogeneity are not relevant to the task of the MMPI. The important criterion, according to Dahlstrom, is not whether an item correlates with other items but whether it improves clinical prediction about patient groups (i.e., external rather than internal validity).

Dahlstrom added that the obvious and subtle dimensions of clinical scales are relatively uncorrelated among normal persons but have much higher correlations for appropriate psychiatric patient reference groups.

As we see here, the issue of the intent of the MMPI is actually irrelevant but for purposes of completeness of the argument, it might be noted that the original purpose of the MMPI may not be as clearcut as Dahlstrom (1969) and Butcher and Tellegen (1978) suggest. Consider the following quotations from the MMPI *Manual* (Hathaway & McKinley, 1951):

> The Minnesota Multiphasic Personality Inventory is a psychometric instrument designed ultimately to provide, in a single test, scores on all the more important phases of personality. The point of view determining the importance of a trait in this case is that of the clinical or personnel worker who wished to assay those traits that are commonly characteristic of disabling psychological abnormality. . . personality characteristics may be assessed on the basis of scores on nine clinical scales originally developed for use with the Inventory. . although the scales are named according to the abnormal manifestation of the symptomatic complex, they have all been shown to have meaning within the normal range. . . as for validity, a high score on a scale has been found to predict positively the corresponding final clinical diagnosis or estimate in more than 60 percent of new psychiatric admissions. (pp. 5-6)

Thus, it appears on the one hand, the constructors of the MMPI are saying that the instrument is intended for differential diagnosis among psychiatric patients and on the other, that scale scores also measure personality characteristics of normal persons.

The most recent edition of the MMPI *Manual* (Hathaway & McKinley, 1983) had less to say about the intent of the instrument, possibly with the thought that it is by now so well known that a statement of purpose is almost gratuitous. The *Manual's* opening sentences state that the MMPI "is designed to provide an objective assessment of some of the major personality characteristics that affect personal and social adjustment. The point of view determining the importance of a trait in this case is that of the clinical or personnel worker who wishes to assay those traits that are commonly characteristic of disabling psychological abnormality " (p.1). No further comment is made beyond this succinct bit of weaseling which still leaves unsettled the not too important issue of whether Hathaway and McKinley intended to create a personality inventory or a diagnostic instrument.

It comes as no great surprise to learn that psychologists working with the MMPI have devised many scales composed of MMPI items. Four different approaches to the development of new measuring instruments from the MMPI pool of 550 items have been employed over the years:

1. Cluster and factor analyses of the total MMPI pool (e.g., Eichman, 1961,1962; Rosen, 1962).

2. Ratios of various clinical scales like the Index of Psychopathology (Sines & Silver, 1963) and the Anxiety Index and Internalization Ratio (Welsh, 1952).

3. Content scales based on selection of items by clinical judgment like the Manifest Anxiety Scale (Taylor, 1953).

4. Empirical selection of items usually based on a comparison of contrasting groups. This procedure has furnished by far the bulk of all the special scales that have been developed from the MMPI pool over the years.

The first edition of Volume I of the MMPI *Handbook* (Dahlstrom & Welsh, 1960) listed 213 special scales and ratios that had been constructed from the MMPI pool. The second edition of this volume (Dahlstrom, Welsh, & Dahlstrom, 1975) contained 455 special scales and ratios. A few years later, Butcher and Tellegen (1978) suggested that there were more special scales than items!

NEGLECT OF THE SPECIAL SCALES

Unfortunately, there is only scanty information on the large majority of special scales. Megargee and Mendelsohn (1962) point out that:

> The clinical researcher who wishes to measure some aspect of personality by using one of these scales often has little information about their real meaning or usefulness. A search of the literature generally reveals little data on which to base a decision for the amount of cross-validation is too often nonexistent or inadequate.Frequently the only information available is that which Dahlstrom and Welsh (1960) have gleaned from unpublished sources, or the title which the scalemaker has given to his instrument. The question natural-ly arises as to how valid these scales are and whether their publication repre-sents progress or merely additional noise in the field. (pp. 431-432)

The development of MMPI special scales often demonstrates "a lack of con-ceptual clarity," according to Clopton (1979a, p.365). He added that this criticism "applies to the naming of newly developed scales, the selection of criterion and comparison groups, and the intended use of the new scale" (p.365). Butcher and Tellegen (1978) note further that:

> Many scales have been contructed by contrasting different "samples of con-venience" (often of heterogeneous makeup or with important characteristics unknown). Often these scales are not cross-validated and more often than not their psychometric properties and inter-relations with other scales are not reported. Many new scales, since they are, after all, derived from the same item pool, prove to be largely redundant alternative versions of existing scales, although sometimes of poorer quality. (p. 622)

Cross-validation or replication is a crucial step in test construction because of the ever-present problem of sampling error and the inevitable possibility of sample bias. If we draw two samples from the same population, we should not expect on purely logical grounds, that *any* MMPI items would significantly differentiate the samples. But it will almost always occur that *some* items, perhaps as many as 5% of them, will indeed be differentially responded to by the two samples. We recog-nize this as a chance occurrence, a function of uncontrolled variables. If we then select a second pair of samples from the same population, we should again expect that about 5% of the items will significantly differentiate the two samples but not by any means the same ones as in the first pair of samples.

In the contrasting groups methods of test construction, the two samples are defined as representing different populations according to some variable or vari-ables: sex, age, race, diagnosis, and so on. But they nonetheless represent the same population with respect to the dependent variable that defines the desired measur-ing instrument (i.e., Sickly Shyness or Robust Extraversion or High Back Pain). Nevertheless, there should be differentiating MMPI items as a sheer function of chance. To test the possibility that this outcome has undermined the test construction, a replication of the investigation is requisite—a cross-validation. If all or most of the original differentiating items are still differentiating in the replication, there is a good chance that a scale has been born. If not, the hypothesis of chance differentiation becomes paramount.

An excellent illustration of cross-validation technique and the need for it is the report by Lachar, Lewis, and Kupke (1979). They administered the MMPI to two small groups of epileptics who were classified as either temporal lobe or nontemporal lobe seizure types on the basis of seizure behavior and electroencephalographic findings. The groups were carefully matched for age, sex, race, education, intelligence, and general neuropsychological impairment. Analysis of the MMPI records revealed no differences between the two groups either on clinical scale scores or 2-point code types.

An item analysis identified 50 MMPI statements which distinguished the two groups. Scores on this set of items, which investigators less cautious than Lachar and his associates might have immediately called the Lobe Identification Scale for Epileptics (LISE), successfully distinguished all members of both groups. Lachar et al. now proceeded to select two new groups of temporal and nontemporal lobe epileptics that were descriptively similar to the original groups. Mean LISE scores obtained by these cross-validation samples were *not* statistically different. The authors conclude that the cross-validation failure "dramatically illustrates the scientific parsimony of successful cross-validation of any new classificatory scale before discussion of its function and item composition" (p. 187).

One can only suspect that a goodly number of the MMPI special scales listed in Dahlstrom et al. (1975) would fail the cross-validation test.

Both Megargee and Mendelsohn and Butcher and Tellegen caution that the title given to a special scale by its constructor may be misleading and should not be accepted uncritically. Again, unfortunately, the large majority of special scales have been inadequately researched to determine whether or not the construct title given to the scale by its constructor is applicable or misleading.

Discussion of the interpretation of special scales is uncommon. Graham (1987), Duckworth and Anderson (1986), and Greene (1980) are exceptions. Graham (1978) has also produced a scholarly review of the experimental findings with a number of the special scales and Clopton (1979a) has contributed a chapter on special scale construction. But there is too much space around these landmarks which doubtlessly explains the limited use of special scales by MMPI diagnosticians (Moreland & Dahlstrom, 1983).

The chronic neglect of the special scale is at least partly due to the conservatism of the major proponents of the MMPI. The usual MMPI workshop perennially presents endless research findings and clinical lore deriving from traditional high-point code typologies. Occasionally, there may be a brief mention of a special scale, usually one that appeared in the old *Basic Readings* compendium (Welsh

& Dahlstrom, 1956). This neglect surely reached a nadir in an article on the future of the MMPI (Faschingbauer, 1979). In this 20-page prophecy, a single 15-word phrase is devoted to special scales!

Even some of those few who take note of the special scales seem to be oppressed by a peculiar ambivalence, perhaps tinged with guilt. Graham (1987), for example, felt obliged to warn his readers in three separate textual admonitions that the special scales "are viewed as supplementary to interpretation of the standard MMPI scales and should not be used instead of these standard scales" (p.116). Duckworth and Anderson (1986), after a dozen years and three editions, have discovered only 14 of the myriad of special scales.

THE PURPOSE OF THIS BOOK

This book is intended to facilitate the clinical employment of MMPI special scales. They offer an abundance of information beyond that provided by the clinical scales and a precision that the clinical scales cannot match. No claim is made that the special scales have ironclad validity. Obviously, they do not, a testimonial to the absence of empirical research. But much the same can be said of high-point codes based on clinical scales. In fact, several large scale investigations strongly suggest that high-point code typologies are sorely lacking in utility (e.g., Palmer, 1970; Huff, 1965; Winters, Weintraub, & Neale, 1981). No solid experimental data supports the conventional high-point code typology. The widely used MMPI code type manuals (e.g., Gilberstadt & Duker, 1965; Marks & Seeman, 1963) are as clinically based as the interpretations offered in this book.

The few proponents of the use of special scales have been candid about the basis of their interpretive suggestions. Duckworth and Anderson (1986), in their chapter on interpretation of special scales, remark that because "little information about them has appeared in the research literature" their interpretations are "based primarily upon our own work in various counseling and clinical settings" (Duckworth & Anderson 1986, p.236). Graham (1987) and Greene (1980) in their MMPI volumes acknowledge "the author's own clinical experience," as Graham put it, as the fundament of special scale analysis.

The interpretations of special scales presented in this volume are also based primarily on clinical experience. What follows is a statement of the source and scope of that experience.

Clinical work with MMPI special scales began at the Indiana University Medical Center in 1969 when Dr. Robert Lushene, then at Florida State University, provided a computer program which scored approximately 115 special scales and ratios in addition to the conventional clinical scales. Over the next 15 years, this program and its several revisions scored somewhere near 70,000 MMPI records derived from more than 75 different populations on 155 scales and ratios. These included not only psychiatric and medical inpatients and outpatients but such diverse groups as applicants for law enforcement agencies, air traffic controllers, the clergy of several religious denominations, parents of children in child psychiatry clinics, applicants for surgical gender reassignment, candidates for various types of positions in industrial and organization settings, and research subjects. Some thousands of these individuals were in direct contact with clinical psychologists at the Indiana University Medical Center, either because the MMPI was part of a test battery, or because the testee was a patient of the psychologist or because the patient was presented as part of a diagnostic or treatment review conference. Some of the agencies outside of the Indiana University Medical Center that made use of the program provided feedback, either systematically or occasionally. All told, a large body of clinical data on a group of more than 150 MMPI special scales was accumulated.[1] Many of them were not found to be useful or to have limited utility. Those scales that have stood the clinical test of time form the fundament of this book. They are listed in Appendix I along with descriptor titles and acronyms.

THE INDIANA SAMPLE

The original Minnesota MMPI normative data are more than four decades old. They may no longer be appropriate, a comment that keeps reappearing in the recent scientific and clinical literature. A major limitation of these norms is that they seem to function most effectively with severely disturbed persons and with respondents who were "demographically most like the original Minnesota normative sample (i.e., white and middle- class)" (Levitt & Duckworth, 1984, p.470). A minor but nagging deficiency is that the 55 items of Scale 5, which are liberally spread among the special scales, were added after the original norming process. No Minnesota normative data are available for these items.

The recent attempt to renorm the MMPI (Colligan,Osborne, Swenson, & Offord, 1983) suggests that a substantial number of items are viewed somewhat differently by contemporary respondents. Colligan et al. provide new norms for the

1   The psychologists who were involved in the aggregation of this pool of information were Frank J. Connolly, Wm. George McAdoo, Nuran B. Miller, and Charles W. Perkins, in addition to the author. Their unwitting but very necessary collaboration with this volume is gratefully acknowledged. Connolly also conceived of the acronym schema for the Harris and Lingoes and the Pepper and Strrong subscales. A large debt to Robert Lushene for his seminal contribution must also be noted with gratitude.

clinical scales and are committed "to extend the tables presented in this reference work to include the most frequently used supplemental scales" (p.286). Unfortunately, the most frequently used special scales, barring a few exceptions, are not the most useful ones so the extension by Colligan and his colleagues may not be particularly fruitful.

It does seem that some kind of normative data for the special scales would be useful. Accordingly, an effort was made to collect a normative data sample in Indiana. The tactic was used by Beck long ago (see Beck, Rabin, Thiesen, Molish, & Thetford, 1950). An entrepreneur kindly makes available his entire staff for testing.[2] These include every literate employee ranging from unskilled laborers, through semi-skilled and skilled workers and office staff to executives. This provided a solid nucleus of 64 respondents. To this group were added 28 adult subjects from research projects and 18 soldiers.[3] Ten of these 110 subjects were discarded because the respondents omitted 30 items or more, or because TR and C1 was at least 5 (see Chapter 2). An effort had been made to have an equal sex ratio but the discarded records left 51 women and 49 men. The demographic characteristics of this sample are shown in Appendix II.

Most of the statistical statements concerning special scales that are made in this book, such as correlations coefficients, are based on the Indiana sample. Appendix III lists means and standard deviations for the various special scales also based on this sample.

Since the Colligan et al. (1983) normative data were collected contemporaneously with the Indiana sample, a comparison of the two sets of data is surely warranted. This comparison is presented in Table 1.2. The data are in the form of K-uncorrected raw scores for Scales 1 through 0 and the conventional validity scales. The census-matched subsample of the Mayo sample, presumably the most unbiased, provided the data in the table. The Indiana and Mayo Clinic data are markedly in accord, especially considering the difference in methodology of data collection and the fact that the Mayo samples were six times as large. The mean absolute difference between the sets of scores for Scales 1 through 0 for males is only 1.64, for females, 1.49. The relatively large differences on Scales 4 and 9 are a function of the age composition of the two samples. The mean ages for males and females in the Mayo census-matched sample were 42.82 and 45.13 compared with 32.2 and 36.2 for the Indiana sample. Subjects over the age of 60 in the Mayo sample scored lowest of all age groups on Scale 4 and 9, certainly nothing unexpected. There were no subjects over age 60 in the Indiana sample.

---

2   The author is deeply indebted to Sidney Tuchman, president of Tuchman Cleaners, for his unique contribution.

3   A similar debt is owed to Major Gary Greenfield, then at Fort Bliss, Texas, for supplying the MMPI records from which the soldier sample was selected.

TABLE 1.2

A Comparison of the Indiana and Mayo Clinic Norms* for the MMPI Clinical and
Validity Scales Using K-Uncorrected Raw Scores

Scale	Males		Females	
	Indiana	Mayo	Indiana	Mayo
1	5.73	5.5	7.24	5.9
2	18.69	18.9	20.35	21.2
3	19.16	20.0	21.16	21.4
4	17.06	15.2	16.63	14.4
5	24.61	20.8	37.08	38.3
6	9.92	9.5	10.14	9.8
7	12.67	11.3	13.20	12.1
8	12.88	10.4	13.04	9.6
9	18.90	15.8	17.65	14.1
0	26.12	27.8	29.75	30.1
Mean Difference		1.64		1.49
L	4.04	3.8	3.82	4.1
F	6.53	4.5	5.27	3.6
K	14.71	14.2	12.75	14.8

*Data from Appendix I in Colligan et al. (1983). The data are for the census-matched subsample

The striking concordance shown in Table 1.2 is shaped by K-correction. This reduces the mean absolute difference to 1.36 for males and 0.61 for females, the latter a function of the fact that the correction wipes out most of the intersample difference on Scales 4 and 9 for females.

The favorable comparison with the Colligan et al. norms suggests a degree of validity for the Indiana sample, despite its small size and unusual composition.

ADOLESCENTS AND MMPI SPECIAL SCALES

It is well established that the evaluation of records of teenaged individuals using adult norms produces seriously exaggerated T-scores on MMPI clinical scales. Archer (1984, 1987), who has twice comprehensively reviewed the literature in this area, summed up by saying that research has "consistently shown that the degree of psychopathology displayed by adolescent respondents tends to be more pronounced when profiles are based on adult norms" (Archer, 1987, p.23).

There is no doubt that Archer is entirely correct. Marks, Seeman, and Haller (1974) plotted mean profiles for large groups of adolescents against the Minnesota adult norms. Male adolescent T-scores on the clinical scales were all above T50, tending to cluster around T60. All of the T-scores on the clinical scales for the female adolescents were above T50 except Scales 1 and 2. The remaining scales tended to cluster around T55. The exaggeration appears to be similar for adolescent inpatients scored by adult norms (Archer, 1987). Five clinical scales for the females and three for the males reached T70 or above. All clinical scales except Scale 0 are at least T60 for both males and females.

Archer (1987) concluded, not unreasonably, that adolescent records should be scored on adolescent norms. The instrumentation to satisfy this excellent advice is unfortunately somewhat lacking for two reasons: (a) Available adolescent clinical scale norms (Hathaway & Monachesi, 1963) are almost as old as the original Minnesota adult norms; and (b) Adolescent norms are available only for a handful of special scales. Gottesman, Hanson, Kroeker, and Briggs (1987) provide norms for 15-year-olds and 18-year-olds on 34 special scales based on the Hathaway and Monachesi (1963) data.

It would be of obvious interest to compare special scale scores obtained by adolescents scored on adult and adolescent norms. The Gottesman et al. adolescent special scale norms have become available so recently that no study employing them has yet appeared in the literature. Immediately available, fortuitously, are special scale data on 100 adolescent female delinquents collected by Haymond (1981). The Haymond sample ranged in age from 12 to 18 with a mean of 15.2. The norms for 15-year-olds furnished by Gottesman et al. would appear to be an appropriate reference group.

Table 1.3 compares 16 of the 34 special scales scored according to T-scores provided by Gottesman et al., the original Minnesota adult norms and the Indiana sample norms. Of the 18 excluded special scales, all have been found not to be clinically useful with the exception of the 2 delinquency scales for which no clinical data are available.

An examination of Table 1.3 indicates clearly that the situation is by no means the same for special scales in adolescent records scored on adult norms as it is for clinical scales. There is definitely no tendency for either the Minnesota or the Indiana adult norms to exaggerate compared to the adolescent norms. Indeed, the Indiana norms appear to *underestimate* the picture yielded by the adolescent norms.

Comparing the adolescent and Minnesota norms, we find that there is an absolute difference on the 16 scales of 4 T-score points. Seven adult scores are above and seven are below the adolescent scale scores. The algebraic difference is zero as indicated in the table.

Of the 15 scales scored by the Indiana norms, 10 are *lower than* their counterparts scored by the adolescent norms. Three are above and two are the same; the absolute difference is 4.07 T-score points and the algebraic difference, as indicated in the table, is -2.1. Nine of the adolescent–Minnesota adult discrepancies and eight of the adolescent–Indiana adult norm discrepancies are 4 T-score points or less.

The data in Table 1.3 strongly suggest that it may be feasible to evaluate adolescent records using special scales applied to adult norms. The case of CI, an

TABLE 1.3
Adolescent Female Delinquents Scored on Adolescent Norms and Two Adult Norms

Scale	Adolescent Norms	Adult Norms	
		Minnesota	Indiana
AUT	62	61	57
DEP	65	61	64
FAM	63	69	61
FEM	43	45	46
HEA	62	55	56
HOS	56	57	56
HYP	53	57	53
MOR	60	55	52
ORG	59	55	53
PHO	53	54	49
PSY	61	67	64
REL	37	47	46
SOC	53	50	48
AMac	58	52	51
D-S	49	49	47
Mean	55.6	55.6	53.5

Note: Adolescent norms provided by Gottesman et al. (1987). Minnesota norms are based on the original standardization sample.

18-year-old, is an excellent illustration (see Chapter 6). The explanation of the sharply different impact of adult norms on the special compared to the clinical scales is a theoretical concern that is beyond comprehensive treatment in this book. One comment: A probable influential factor is that in the clinical scale comparative investigations, the clinical scales were, as usual, K-corrected. Special scales are never K-corrected.

Nevertheless, the clinician should exercise caution in using adult norms for adolescent records. The analyses of Table 1.3 encompass only a handful of the variety of special scales that are available and not all special scales will necessarily yield the same result as the Wiggins' Scales, AMac, and D-S. For example, clinical use clearly indicates that for 9PMA, adult norms would result in serious overestimations of adolescent records. Normal adolescents score around T70 on the average when adult norms are applied.

On the positive side, one might very well expect that the differences in Table 1.3 would be even less for a sample of normal adolescents since by all indications, psychopathology in teenagers tends to increase the distortion produced by the application of adult norms.

CHAPTER 2
THE VALIDITY SCALES

The creators of the MMPI were aware of the fakability of a verbal inventory. They attempted to develop several validity indicators, internal measures that would point to the individual who was not responding honestly. As it happens, none of these scales is a reliable identifier of the dishonest respondent, though the regular employment of at least one of them—the F Scale—continues. The hardiness of this measure is partly a function of some confusion about the term, *invalidity*. The question is: Valid for what purpose? A scale that elevates when the respondent is badly confused or psychotic suggests that the record may be invalid as personality assessment. Since it assists in diagnosis, it does not indicate that the record is invalid as a diagnostic device.

TRADITIONAL VALIDITY MEASURES

Although less widely known and used than the original MMPI indices, there are three measures that are more effective signallers of the potentially invalid record. Before presenting them, a brief review of the known inadequacies of the earlier scales seems warranted.

Lie Scale

The Lie (L) Scale was contructed by the developers of the MMPI on a completely nonempirical, rational basis. It consists of 15 statements whose context is such that a truthful respondent would be highly likely to respond "True" to every statement. Here are some illustrations of these items.

> I do not always tell the truth.
> I do not like everyone I know.
> I would rather win than lose a game.

The intent of the L Scale is that it should provide "a measure of the degree to which the subject may be attempting to falsify his scores by always choosing the response that places him in the most acceptable light socially" (Hathaway & Mc-Kinley, 1951, p.18). Unfortunately, the gambit is too obvious to anyone of at least average intelligence, a view that is consensually shared by clinicians. An investigation by Lebovits and Ostfeld (1967) not unexpectedly showed that L Scale scores and educational level are negatively correlated.

Yet, almost no one *always* makes the socially acceptable response to the L Scale. Gravitz (1970) collected records of more than 11,000 young adults and found only five L Scale items that came close to the "always" criterion (90% false responses). The deviant (true) response was chosen for four items by more than 50% of the respondents. Hathaway and McKinley (1951) themselves concluded that raw score of 7 on the L Scale was "probably very significant" and would "require interpretation, although not necessarily implying a priori invalidity of the findings" (p.23).

The L Scale is also insensitive to certain response sets. An individual who endorsed every item would be identified by the maximum L Scale score of 15. But a person who responded "false" to every item would receive a score of 0 and the respondent who alternatingly gave true and false responses would obtain a score of 6, still in the acceptable range according to Hathaway and McKinley.

Occasionally, the L Scale may trap a respondent with his or her best foot forward. The victim is likely to be below the average range of intelligence and with less than a 12th-grade education. But even this isolated case must be examined carefully because high L Scores, although they have little to do with validity of the record, do have meaning and may be interpretable in a different framework. The use of the L Scale as a personality measure is discussed in a subsequent chapter.

F Scale

The F Scale is one of the most misunderstood and misused subsections of the MMPI. It is composed of 64 items that evoked responses in the deviant direction by 10% or less of the segment of the Minnesota standardization sample that was collected prior to 1940. The F Scale was intended as a check on the validity of the record. A high score supposedly indicated that "the other scales are likely to be invalid either because the subject was careless or unable to comprehend the items or because extensive scoring or recording errors were made." A low F score is a "reliable indication that the subject's responses were rational and relatively pertinent" (Hathaway & McKinley, 1951, p.18). The detection of "faking bad" was not originally mentioned as a purpose for the F Scale but it has certainly been used for this purpose (e.g., Graham, 1987).

Examination of the item content of the F Scale suggests that a number of the items were poorly chosen if the intent was to measure deviancy apart from psychopathology. Thirteen of the items—20% of the total—deal with hallucinations and delusions. Fifteen of the items are found on Scale 8 and nine are found on Scale 6. Not surprisingly, the unweighted mean correlation between the F Scale and Scale 8 in nine investigations was .69; with Scale 6, .37 (Dahlstrom et al., 1975). In the two studies that utilized outpatients, the unweighted mean correlations were respectively .80 and .55.

There is almost no overlap between the F Scale and Scale 7, yet the unweighted mean correlation for the nine investigations was .46; for the two patient samples alone, .63 (Dahlstrom et al., 1975).

Greene (1980) provided an excellent review of the experimental work that demonstrates the relationship between the F Scale and psychopathology. He summed up by noting that patients with raw F Scale scores of 23 or more are "likely to be severely disorganized and psychotic; these characteristics are readily apparent in an interview" (p.40). Greene might have added that scores of this magnitude are extremely rare in other than patient groups.

Thus, there seems to be little question that the F Scale measures psychopathology as a form of deviancy. It is entirely questionable whether it measures invalidity as deviancy.

The original MMPI norms are probably no longer entirely appropriate. However, in dealing with scales, since they are collections of items, the error that is made in using the original norms may not be serious. For example, it probably would not matter much that a T-score of 70 on Scale 3 should be 30 instead of 28. But this is not true in dealing with individual items. Thus, the validity of the F Scale is further compromised by the fact that contemporaneously, some of the items might no longer be endorsed in the deviant direction by less than 10% of a normative sample. The data of Colligan et al.(1983) suggest that eight items in the F Scale currently have endorsement in the deviant direction by substantially greater than 10% of the respondents (items 14, 20, 112, 115, 164, 199, 206, and 215). For example, averaging data for males and females, the deviant response to the items "I am very religious (more than most people)," "I have used alcohol excessively," and "My sex life is satisfactory," was given by about 20% of Colligan's modern sample.

Respondents wishing to "fake bad," that is, to exaggerate their psychopathology, usually endorse obvious items that admit to symptoms of anxiety and depression. There are few such items on the F Scale. Nearly 40% of the items are psychotic manifestations or peculiar or unusual postures, mostly antisocial and criminal behaviors. Such items are seldom employed by respondents seeking to fake bad. Responses to the largest group of items—about one third—would clearly be socially deviant but again, these are not emotional symptom items of the type commonly used to fake bad. On this basis alone, it is doubtful that the F Scale is a satisfactory measure of faking bad unless the respondent wished to present himself/herself as overly psychotic. To be sure, such individuals can be found among forensic patients but since the spuriously elevated F Scale will be paralleled by elevated Scales 6 and/or 7 and/or 8, it is difficult to see that the F Scale itself contributes. The typical "cry for help" individual does not usually fake bad with psychotic items and is less likely to be detected by the F Scale.

To summarize, the F Scale is not recommended as an index of validity in the clinical assessment situation although it maybe properly employed to discard inappropriate subjects in experiments.

K Scale

The original purpose of this scale was to identify "defensiveness against psychological weakness, and . . . . a defensiveness that verges upon deliberate distortion in the direction of making a more 'normal' appearance" (Hathaway & McKinley, 1951, p.18). In other words, the respondent who scores high on K is engaging either in denial in the psychodynamic sense or is just plain lying.

The derivation of the K Scale leaves much to be desired. The selection of items was based essentially on a group of 50 psychiatric inpatients all of whom obtained MMPI clinical scale profiles (uncorrected by K, of course) that had no scale above a T-Score of 70. A second qualification was that each had an L Scale T-score of at least 60. The idea, of course, was that such individuals, who were identified as seriously ill by reason of hospitalization, were being defensive because of their MMPI records. This assumption has two deficiencies. First, an individual with K- uncorrected T-Scores on clinical scales that are in the 60 to 69 range may be manifesting considerable psychopathology. Second, the L Scale is a poor measure of test-taking defensiveness.

To begin with, a problem arises in the identification of denial as a unconscious mechanism. Denial, like other defense mechanisms, can exist on a psychotic or neurotic level but it can also be an adaptive strategy. Indeed, denial is probably the most common defense mechanism used by normal people (Levitt, 1980b). Is the high K scorer very ill or deliberately lying or symptom-free? Greene (1980) suggested that the K Scale measures normality among normal persons and defensiveness among the maladjusted. The distinction has little empirical backing but in any event, the population to which the respondent belongs is very often unknown. Indeed, the very purpose of the administration of the MMPI may be to determine the population to which the respondent belongs.

Examination of the K Scale items suggests a more lengthy L Scale. It is not difficult to perceive that a normal person who responded truthfully to the best of his/her comprehension, could obtain a raw score from 15 to 25, corresponding to T-Scores of 78 and 98 in the Minnesota norms. It also seems evident that an individual who is defending himself/herself against awareness of a negative self-concept could obtain a high score. It also seems possible that individuals with behavior disorders (principal component of the original 50 cases) might obtain a high score through malingering.

In summary, the K Scale does not appear to be useful as a validity measure either on the basis of theoretical considerations or empirical research.

F minus K Index

Combining the F and K Scales as a validity indicator was proposed by Gough (1950). The idea, of course, is that if F is substantially higher than K, then the respondent is faking bad, trying to exaggerate psychopathology. If the K is so much greater than F, then the respondent was being defensive.

There is no reason to expect that F minus K would be any more effective as a validity indicator than either of its components individually and indeed this seems to be the case. The relevant literature has again been succinctly summed up by Greene (1980). In general, F minus K is at best inconsistent in identifying test-taking attitudes, especially faking bad. It does not function any more effectively in identifying faking bad profiles than does F alone. The union of F and K is no more successful as a validity indicator than either of its components alone and its clinical use is not recommended.

Omitted Items (Qu)

When measurement requires that the subject respond either true or false to a fixed number of items, simple common sense indicates that the accuracy of assessment will be impaired if the subject fails to respond to some number of items. Evaluation of the damage as a function of the frequency of omissions is no simple matter.

The number of items to which the subject had failed to respond, Qu, or represented schematically as ?, was one of the the first ideas about validity that occurred to the developers of the MMPI.

The concept itself was obviously unchallengeable but the number of omitted items that should invalidate a record completely was unknown nor did Hathaway and McKinley have any sound method of making this determination. The use of T-scores made no sense. The Minnesota normative sample omitted a mean of 2.83 items with an SD of 1.5. The omission of a little more than 1% of the inventory's items would hardly seem to invalidate a record. Instead, Hathaway and McKinley suggested quite arbitrarily that a Qu above 30 should be viewed with suspicion.

A fair amount of evidence shows that except for a population that is defined by serious deficiency in reading comprehension or by intellectual deficit, no group averages more than a Qu of 5. The mean for the Indiana normative sample was 1.77. While such a finding is of interest, it does not really help in establishing a cut-off point for record invalidity based on omitted items.

A study by Clopton and Neuringer (1979) assessed the impact of omitted items on high-point codes. They found that a little more than 25% of code types were altered by the omission of 30 items. Looking at the other side, more than 40% of the high-point codes were unchanged by the omission of as many as 120 items. The applied significance of this study is unclear but in any event, it has no reference for the clinician who is diagnosing with special scales rather than clinical scales.

Invalidity due to item omission is not a serious problem for the MMPI clinician as long as he/she is aware of the intellectual impact on test validity. It requires about a seventh- grade reading level to be able to complete the MMPI validly (Ward & Ward, 1980). Among those who do not have intellectual problems, clinical experience indicates that less than 1 in 20 will have a Qu of 10 or above. The most commonly omitted items are those about which many people feel uncertain such as "I believe in a life hereafter." Four items that were omitted by more than 10% of the original Minnesota normal group dealt with religious beliefs: 58, 98, 249, and 483 (Dahlstrom et al., 1975). Others deal with circumstances in which the respondent could not have an opinion because of lack of experience such as "When I was a child I liked to play hopscotch" or "I like to read mechanics magazines."Occasionally, items are inadvertently omitted.

While it is true that records are affected by omitted items, they are almost never totally invalidated. Any scale that is elevated despite omissions is all the more significant for that reason. It is more important for the clinician to know which items have been omitted than how many. A cluster of omitted items dealing with the same matter such as family problems or sexual behavior has evident clinical significance. The single omitted item in the case of SV presented in Chapter 6 was a diagnostic clue.

THE NEWER VALIDITY MEASURES

Test-Retest (TR)

Sixteen of the 550 items of the MMPI are duplicated on the first response sheet that was developed for group administration of the inventory. The purpose was to facilitate machine scoring, nothing more. This 566-item form persists even though the replicated 16 items are no longer necessary for scoring purpose. Indeed, it is not at all uncommon to find the MMPI described as an instrument composed of 566 items.

The idea of using the replicated items as a check on the validity of the record was originally suggested by Buechley and Ball (1952). The assumption is that in the valid record, each item in each pair of replicated items will receive the same response. To the extent that responses to the same item are not the same across the 16 pairs, invalidity is suggested. Scores on TR can range from 0 to 16 although Buechley and Ball, for convenience, worked with only 14 pairs of items.

This tactic was later adopted deliberately by Edwards (1959) in the development of his Personal Preference Schedule. He termed the number of agreements among pairs of identical items as a *consistency score*.

Buechley and Ball believed that the major source of invalidity among MMPI records was random responding, probably a function of lack of motivation and unwillingness to bother to read and to try to understand. This does occur among patients and subjects occasionally but clinical experience suggests that two other conditions more often account for elevated TR scores: confusion and poor reading ability or verbal comprehension. Great haste in responding, leading to carelessness, is another possible source of high TR scores.

Bond (1986), on the basis of his research, has proposed that the primary force behind the TR score is simply indecision and thus its utility as a measure of invalidity is questionable. Indecisiveness is more likely to be a causal factor among Bond's normal college student subjects than it is among patient groups. Bond's data suggest that TR should be applied cautiously with normal subjects who have adequate reading skills.

Table 2.1 gives some T-scores on various relevant measures for three individuals who scored high on TR. Subject A was an adult male outpatient. The MMPI had been administered to him shortly after his arrest on a morals charge, a moment when he was extremely emotionally upset. Note that the F Scale would not have identified this man's confusion.

A record was obtained from this patient a few weeks later when he was reasonably calm (A^2). The changes in the various measures would be expected in accordance with the reduced TR score.

Subjects B and C were inmates of a correctional institution for delinquent girls. B admitted after taking the test that she regarded it as too much trouble and had

Table 2.1

Three Cases Illustrating the Use of TR

Case	State	Sex	Age	TR	F	K	ME
A	Confusion	Male	39	8	62	30	68
A²	Not Confused			0	48	56	61
B	Random Responding	Female	15	9	100	48	70
C	Poor verbal comprehension	Female	15	9	125	64	79

responded without bothering to read the items. Posttest inquiry disclosed that Subject C's verbal comprehension was insufficient to complete the inventory validly even though the MMPI was administered on tape. Note that while F identified both girls, so did ME, the average T-score for eight clinical scales.

Buechley and Ball reported a mean TR of 2.8 for a group of male delinquents. This is in accord with a mean of 2.6 found by Haymond (1981) with delinquent girls. The mean TR for the Indiana sample before removing records with TR of 4 and above was 1.27. The mean for the males was 0.75, for the females, 1.75. This difference is statistically significant ($t = 2.88, p < .01$), suggesting that cutting scores for TR should vary by sex.

Buechley and Ball proposed a cut-off score of 3 to identify the invalid record, equivalent to T59 in the total Indiana sample. This seems a bit too conservative. In the Indiana sample, T70 would be equivalent to a raw score of almost 4 for the males and between 5 and 6 for the females. Reasonable cutting scores would appear to be 4 for males and 5 (T66) for females.

Carelessness Scale

TR is a more effective validity indicator than the F Scale on both logical and empirical grounds. Greene (1978, 1980) has pointed out that TR does have one shortcoming. It cannot identify the individual who responds True to every MMPI item or who responds False to every item. Such respondents are rare but they would be missed by TR which would, of course, give them a score of 0.

Greene (1979) devised the Carelessness Scale (Cl) as a validity indicator that did not miss the all-True and all-False respondents. Cl consists of 12 pairs of items, 7 of which should be answered in the same direction on logical grounds and 5 of which should be answered in an opposite direction. Whichever way a thoughtful, clear-headed individual responds to the item, "Most of the time I feel blue," he/she should respond opposite to the item, "I am happy most of the time." Responses to the items, "I am never happier than when I am alone," and "I dislike having people about me," should be the same, whether true or false.

The methodology of the development of Cl (Greene, 1978) is somewhat un-clear. The MMPI contains may item pairs that should logically elicit responses that are either the same or opposite. On inspection, some of Greene's pairs do not seem well chosen. For example, it appears quite possible to be "afraid to be alone in the dark" and yet not to be "often afraid of the dark." More than one respondent in four in Greene's (1978) three samples gave the deviant (different) response to the item pair, "I am very seldom troubled by constipation," and "I have had no dif-ficulty in starting or holding my bowel movements." The degree of deviancy may be a function of ambiguity of the expression "holding" a bowel movement.

Nevertheless, the scale works out fairly well in clinical practice, especially in tandem with TR. Like a high score on TR, a high score on Cl suggests that the respondent either was confused at the time that the inventory was administered, or lacks sufficient reading comprehension to complete the inventory validly.

Greene (1978, 1980) noted that his patient groups on whom Cl was developed obtained mean Cl scores of 1.76 and 2.20 while a college student sample mean was 1.48. In the Indiana normative sample, the mean C1 was 1.59 with an SD of 1.29 which fits with Greene's normal subjects. Greene (1980) proposed that a score of 4 is "indeterminate" while a score of 5 is definitely "inconsistent." A score of 4 would be equivalent to T69 in the Indiana sample distribution and 5 would be T76. The decision is most effectively made in conjunction with TR. When TR is 2 or less for males, or 3 or less for females, C1 should be at least 5 to consider invalidity. If TR is greater than 2 for males or greater than 3 for females, a Cl of 4 is sufficient for the consideration of invalidity.

Mean Elevation (ME)

One of the early research reports on the MMPI (Modlin, 1947) suggested that the average elevation of the nine scales then in existence (including Scale 5 but not Scale 0) could be used as a rough index of psychopathology. Modlin believed that an average elevation of 70 or above (uncorrected for K which was not proposed as a correction until 1948) indicated "major pathology."

No one appears to have taken seriously Modlin's notion that an agglomeration of MMPI clinical scales scores "might be employed as a screening questionnaire or psychosomatic index," and its use as a general index is infrequently reported (e.g., Cernovsky, 1986). The nature of the faking bad profile does, however, suggest a potential use for the average elevation of the clinical scales (ME). Since Scale 0 is most often uninvolved in the faking bad tactic, the diagnostic capacity of ME is sharpened by basing it on the remaining eight scales.

It is generally agreed that the vast majority of MMPI clinical profiles can be classified as having a "high-point pair" as Greene (1980) labeled it, or high-point code, in the conventional parlance. In the psychiatric patient, the high points may be expected to exceed T70. Other scale elevations might reasonably range from T55 to T69. In a large majority of records, this distribution would yield an ME below T70.

For example, two scales at T75, four scales at T65 and two at T60 would produce an ME of 66. Even if the high-point pair was at T80, ME would be below 68.

However, it is difficult to attain an ME of 75 without diffuse elevation of the clinical scales. For example, even if the high-point pair was at T90, the remaining scales would have to average 70 in order to come out with an ME of 75. Even with three scales at T90, the remaining scales would need to average 66. With three scales at T80, the remaining scales must average 72 in order to yield an ME of 75.

In the Indiana normative sample, ME with K-corrected clinical scales was 58.32 for males and 56.00 for females with corresponding SD's of 5.94 and 6.35. (For K-uncorrected scales, the respective means were 49.02 and 49.01.) In these distributions, T75 lies three standard deviations above the mean, an interesting coincidence. Like other validity indicators, the variance of ME has no applied meaning.

Clinical experience suggests that records with an ME of 75 or more for eight K-corrected clinical scales, or 70 or more for K-uncorrected scales, are likely to have been obtunded by confusion, serious reading disability, acute psychosis or a faking bad response set.

CHAPTER 3
SOME USEFUL SPECIAL
SCALES

THE HARRIS AND LINGOES SUBSCALES
OF THE CLINICAL SCALES

Almost from the birth of the MMPI, it has been evident that its clinical scales are multidimensional and that those scales are by no means the only possible effective measuring instruments that could be extracted from the 550 item MMPI pool. An early attempt to capitalize on the multidimensionality were the subscales developed by Harris and Lingoes (1955, rev. 1968). They attempted to formulate dimensionally homogeneous subscales from each of the clinical scales using their combined clinical judgment. Apparently, the strategy was a conference technique since no interrater reliabilities were ever reported.

A total of 31 subscales were created from six clinical scales; the items in Scales 1 and 7 did not "lend themselves to classification" according to Harris and Lingoes (1955, rev. 1968). Table 3.1 lists the subscales with their respective descriptions and acronyms.

Subscales derived from Scales 2, 3, 6, and 9 have minimal item overlap except for 2B (D5) which is entirely contained within 2SD (D1). Subscale 4A (Pd4) is the sum of 4SOA (Pd4A) and 4SEA (Pd4B). Subscale 8IPA (Sc2) is a composite of 8COG (Sc2A), 8CON (Sc2B), and 8DIC (Sc2C). The three composite scales are generally not regarded as useful so that the Harris and Lingoes subscales are considered to number 28.

The Harris and Lingoes scales are employed in clinical situations to some unknown extent. Unfortunately, as Greene (1980) pointed out, research with these scales, especially investigations bearing on validity, is scanty. A statistical study by Lingoes himself (1960) suggested only that factor analyzing the Harris and Lingoes scales results in at least seven factors and possibly as many as 14. An earlier

Table 3.1

THE HARRIS & LINGOES SUBSCALES OF THE MMPI CLINICAL SCALES

H & L Designation	H & L Descriptor	Acronym
D 1	Subjective Depression	2 S D
D 2	Psychomotor Retardation	2 P R
D 3	Physical Malfunctioning	2 P M
D 4	Mental Dullness	2 M D
D 5	Brooding	2 B
H y 1	Denial of Social Anxiety	3DSA
H y 2	Need for Affection	3NA
H y 3	Lassitude-Malaise	3LM
H y 4	Somatic Complaints	3SC
H y 5	Inhibition of Aggression	3IA
P d 1	Familial Discord	4 F D
P d 2	Authority Conflict	4 A C
P d 3	Social Imperturbability	4 S I
P d 4	Alienation	4 A
P d 4 a	Social Alienation	4 S O A
P d 4 b	Self-alienation	4 S E A
P a 1	Paranoid Ideation	6PI
P a 2	Poignancy	6P
P a 3	Naivete	6N
S c 1	Object Loss	8 O L
S c 1 a	Social Alienation	8 S O A
S c 1 b	Emotional Alienation	8 E A
S c 2	Intrapsychic Autonomy	8 I P A
S c 2 a	Lack of Ego-Mastery, Cognitive	8 C O G
S c 2 b	Lack of Ego-Mastery, Conative	8 C O N
S c 2 c	Lack of Ego-Mastery, Defect of Inhibition & Control	8 D I C
S c 3	Bizarre Sensory Experiences	8 B S E
M a 1	Amorality	9 A M O
M a 2	Psychomotor Acceleration	9 P M A
M a 3	Imperturbability	9 I M P
M a 4	Ego Inflation	9 E I

investigation by Panton (1959) did no more than provide norms for a prison population.

There has been at least one full-scale attempt to examine the criterion validity of the Harris and Lingoes scales (Calvin, 1975). It has a number of methodological shortcomings among which is the sample—all mental patients—that limit inferences that could be drawn from the data. Nevertheless, this study is so rare that it is worthy of commentary.

Calvin set up seven criteria, some of which were clinically based such as diagnosis and patient's attitude toward a significant other as reported by the significant other and by the patient, and the patient's view of his/her reason for admission. Some were less clinical but still hardly objective; the 30-item Nurses Observation Scale for Inpatient Evaluation (NOSIE) and the Gorham Brief Psychiatric Rating Scale (GBPRS) which is based on a psychiatric interview. Neither the NOSIE nor the GBPRS are intended for research and there are no interrater reliabilities in this investigation. Since the NOSIE has 30 items which were used individually by Calvin, there was actually a total of 37 possible criterion measures for any particular

Harris and Lingoes scale. The actual number of criteria for a scale varied from as many as 10 to as few as 2, but none was a really firm, objective standard. Calvin himself determined the criteria for each scale, another weakness of this investigation.

Essentially, Calvin found that the Harris and Lingoes subscales on the whole tended to have approximately the same criterion validity as their respective clinical scales. Thus, according to Calvin, "very little is added" to the interpretation of a clinical scale by its Harris and Lingoes subscales. This appears to be true for Scales 2, 6, and 8 which did rather well with their criterion measures. Scales 3, 4, and 9 did more poorly in relating to criteria. The subscales of these clinical scales may be worth noting, although Calvin did not seem to think so. Thus, 3NA (Hy2), 3SC (Hy4), 4FD (Pd1), 4AC (Pd2), and 9IMP (Ma3) were all significantly related to criteria to a greater extent than their respective clinical scales.

Calvin's data are useful in that they reflect some degree of validity for some of the Harris and Lingoes scales. His research, however, does not impinge on a major utility of the Harris and Lingoes scale, i.e., the determination of the cause of a significant elevation of a clinical scale. Because of the multidimensionality of the clinical scales, a respondent may have an elevated score on Scale 3 without symptoms of dissociation; on Scale 4 without being rebellious; on Scale 6 without being paranoid, on Scale 8 without being psychotic, and on Scale 9 without being manic. The subscales assist in determining whether such conclusions are valid. This was the original intent of Harris and Lingoes (1955): the subscales were to be "an aid to profile interpretation." Graham (1978) and Clopton (1979a) have made reference to this original intent and it doubtlessly is the more common utilization of these groupings of items.

What follows are three cases that illustrate this employment of the Harris and Lingoes scales. They were not chosen at random but neither are they atypical. Such cases constitute about 25% of all records, a higher percentage of patient records.

Case D65 has a peak on Scale 6 (Figure 3.1). The Harris and Lingoes subscales of Scale 6 indicate that this elevation is not due to manifest paranoid ideation: 6PI is not seriously elevated. Also, this respondent endorsed no items on the Indiana Severe Reality Distortions Scale (I-RD) which is composed of all the delusion and hallucination items in the MMPI pool. The other subscales indicate that the Scale 6 elevation is due primarily to the subject's view of herself as a moral, virtuous individual and one who tends to be somewhat naive (6N - Pa3). The elevation is also a function of some tendency to be hypersensitive (6P-Pa2). These attributes do not add up to a paranoid tendency in the classical sense. One must allow that there are a number of normal women in the community who are naive, somewhat hypersensitive and regard themselves as virtuous.

Case AA38 is a 4-3 but the elevation on the latter scale will stand examination (Figure 3.2). The Harris and Lingoes subscales of Scale 3 show clearly that

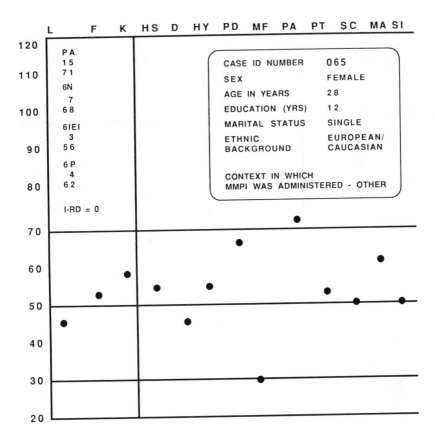

Figure 3.1 Profile of case D65

an important share of the elevation on that scale is due to 3LM (Hy3) a group of physical symptoms frequently associated with anxiety and depression. Equally importantly, this respondent failed to endorse a single item on the Indiana Dissociative Symptoms Scale (I-DS) which is composed of all the dissociative symptoms in the MMPI pool. In summary, the elevation on Scale 3 does not represent hysterical tendencies in the usual sense but is a function of the fact that this respondent has endorsed a significant number of physical symptom items. Obviously, it is perfectly possible for an individual to have health concerns without being a hysterical personality or even having hysteroid tendencies.

Case D54 is the supposedly paradoxical 4-7, more than usually worthy of scrutiny of the subscales (Figure 3.3). It happens that D54 is socially anxious rather than socially poised-4SI (Pd3) is quite low—her scores are within normal limits on 4SOA (Pd4a), a scale which measures the tendencies to externalize blame, to feel put upon by society and so on, and on 4AC (Pd2), the expression of hostility and

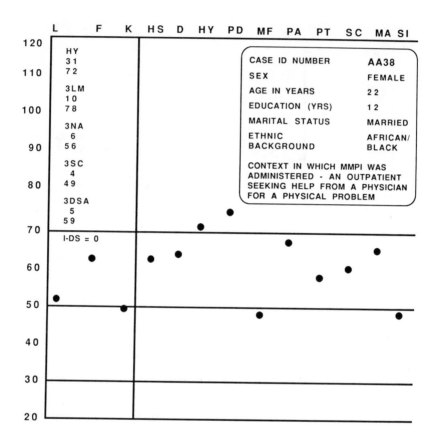

Figure 3.2 Profile of case AA38

rebelliousness. Much of the elevation on Scale 4 is evidently a function of 4SEA (Pd4b) which is composed of a series of depression-like items that describe dissatisfaction with the self rather than the environment, not at all consonant with the conventional interpretation of a high 4.

The tendency for the Harris and Lingoes subscales to follow along with their respective clinical scales has also been reported by Moos and Solomon (1964) and Lebovits, Visotsky, and Ostfeld (1960). As in the Calvin study, there were a few exceptions.

Lebovits et al. administered the MMPI during hallucinogenic experience for a small group of subjects serving as their own control. The subscale changes of interest that occurred were a decrease in 3NA (Hy2) and an increase in 3LM (Hy3)

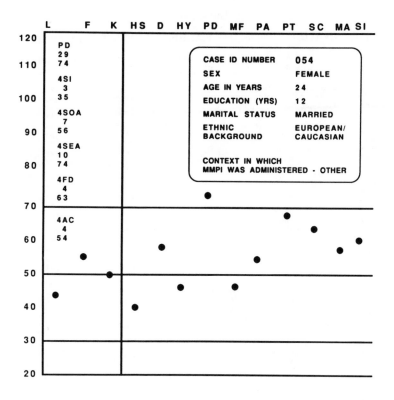

Figure 3.3 Profile of case D54

compared to normal state despite the fact that Scale 3 did not show any interstate difference.

Moos and Solomon compared a group of rheumatoid arthritics with a group of their family members as a control. Again, most of the subscale differences followed clinical scale differences with the notable exception of 8CON (Sc2b) which was significantly elevated in the arthritic group although Scale 8 itself was not. 8CON is a measure of general motivation, of elan for life, an understandable deficiency in these patients although they are evidently not psychotic.

Individual Harris and Lingoes subscales have occasionally appeared in experimental work. McCreary (1975) compared groups of child molesters with and without a record of prior arrests. The arrested group scored significantly higher on Scale 4 but much of the difference was due to a highly significant difference on 4AC (Pd2). In contrast, 4FD (Pd1) showed hardly even an absolute difference be-

Table 3.2

CLINICAL EVALUATION OF THE HARRIS & LINGOES SUBSCALES

H & L Designation	Acronym	H & L Descriptor	Number of Items	Item Homogeneity	Appropriate Label	Clinical Utility
D 1	2SD	Subjective Depression	32	yes	yes	fair
D 2	2PR	Psychomotor Retardation	15	yes	yes	good
D 3	2PM	Physical Malfunctioning	11	yes	yes	fair
D 4	2MD	Mental Dullness	15	yes	yes	good
D 5	2B	Brooding	10	no	no	poor
Hy1	3DSA	Denial of Social Anxiety	6	yes	yes	good
Hy2	3NA	Need for Affection	12	yes	yes	good
Hy3	3LM	Lassitude-Malaise	15	yes	yes	fair
Hy4	3SC	Somatic Complaints	17	yes	yes	fair
Hy5	3IA	Inhibition of Aggression	7	no	no	poor
Pd1	4FD	Familial Discord	9	yes	yes	good
Pd2	4AC	Authority Conflict	8	yes	yes	good
Pd3	4SI	Social Imperturbability	12	yes	yes	good
Pd4	4A	Alienation	24	no	no	poor
Pd4a	4SOA	Social Alienation	18	yes	yes	good
Pd4b	4SEA	Self-alienation	15	yes	no	fair
Pa1	6PI	Ideas of External Influence	17	yes	yes	fair
Pa2	6P	Poignancy	9	yes	no	good
Pa3	6AMV	Affirmation of Moral Virtue	9	yes	yes	good
Sc1	8OL	Object Loss	32	no	no	poor
Sc1a	8SOA	Social Alienation	21	yes	yes	good
Sc1b	8EA	Emotional Alienation	11	yes	no	fair
Sc2	8IPA	Intra-psychic Autonomy	35	no	no	poor
Sc2a	8COG	Lack of Ego-Mastery, Cognitive	10	yes	yes	good
Sc2b	8CON	Lack of Ego-Mastery, Conative	14	yes	yes	good
Sc2c	8DIC	Lack of Ego-Mastery, Defect of Inhibition and Control	11	no	yes	poor
Sc3	8BSE	Bizarre Sensory Experiences	20	yes	yes	fair
Ma1	9AMO	Amorality	6	yes	yes	good
Ma2	9PMA	Psychomotor Acceleration	11	yes	yes	good
Ma3	9IMP	Imperturbability	8	yes	yes	good
Ma4	9EI	Ego Inflation	9	no	no	poor

tween the two groups. Unfortunately, the remainder of the Harris and Lingoes subscales of Scale 4 are not presented.

3IA (Hy5) failed to distinguish between groups of violent and nonviolent yong adult male criminals in a report by Lothstein and Jones (1978). This is one of the Harris and Lingoes subscales that is mislabeled and not useful so this negative finding is not surprising.

Subscale 3IA is one of a number of Harris and Lingoes scales that are mislabeled, have heterogenous item content, have too few items to be directly useful, or have other defects. Table 3.2 presents an analysis of the Harris and Lingoes scales, indicating those that have defects and those that are useful and not useful.

Examination of the item content of the Harris and Lingoes scales discloses that several are clearly heterogenous collections of items that do not appear to belong to the same family. These include 2B (D5), 3IA (Hy5), 8DIC (Sc2c), 8OL (Sc1), and 9EI (Ma4). The titles of 2B, 3IA and 9EI appear to derive from a single item in the subscale. 8DIC (Sc2C) indeed covers what might be broadly termed *defects of inhibition and control*. However, its items deal with a number of individual areas causing loss of control such as dissociation, tension, mania, hypersensitivity, paranoia, and phobia. This heterogeneity makes it all but impossible to interpret a high score on this subscale.

Other subscales also seem to have been mislabeled. This is not particularly surprising. Butcher and Tellegen (1978) once remarked that "new MMPI scales, like many of the old ones, should not be assumed to measure the characteristics suggested by its name or by its author"(p.623). Harris and Lingoes (1968) themselves cautiously claimed "no particular brief" for their subscale titles and noted that others "would undoubtedly have assigned different names" (p.1).

Subscales 4SEA (Pd4b) and 8EA (Sc1b) have item homogeneity but are labeled misleadingly. Both are composed primarily of depression items like "Most of the time I feel blue," "I believe I am a condemned person" and "I am happy most of the time (False)." This explains why these two measures had loadings ranging from .70 to .86 on a Depression factor for both sexes in the three patient populations tested by Foerstner (1986) in her factor analytic study of MMPI special scales. These mini-depression scales are inferior to depression scales developed by Wiggins (1966) and by Tryon, et al. (Tryon, 1966; Stein, 1968).

Much the same criticism can be made for subscales dealing with health concerns: 2PM (D3), 3LM (Hy3), and 3SC (Hy4). While these serve to separate out the physical symptom aspects of Scales 2 and 3, they contain too few items to be directly useful clinically. Other special scales, notably Wiggins' Poor Health (HEA) and Organic Symptoms (ORG) scales and the Tryon, Stein, and Chu Body Symptom scale (TSC/B) are more effective measures of health concerns. Similarly, half of the items on 8BSE (Sc3) are duplicated on Wiggins' Organic Symptoms scale (ORG) which is the superior index of the claim of dissociative/ neurological symptoms because of its greater item constituency. On occasion, a smaller health concerns scale elevates while a larger one does not, a circumstance that is worth investigating by direct examination of item content.

Fifteen of the Harris and Lingoes subscales have been found to be clinically useful in themselves. They are listed in Table 3.3 along with their clinically based interpretations.

Table 3.3

CLINICAL INTERPRETATIONS OF SELECTED HARRIS & LINGOES SUBSCALES

Subscale	Interpretation
2PR (D2)	High scorers claim to lack sufficient energy to carry on routine activities. When other depression indices are high, a low score on this scale points to a suicide potential.
2MD (D4)	High scorers feel that they are beset by cognitive difficulties; including inability to reason clearly, to make decisions, to think logically. Memory is also impaired.
3DSA (Hy1)	Low scorers tend to be socially maladroit and anxious, shy, embarrass easily and are generally uncomfortable in social situations. This scale clusters with 4SI (Pd3) and 9LMP (Ma3). High scorers are socially comfortable. Respondents scoring above T70 may be reflecting denial.
4SI (Pd3)	See 3DSA.
4AC (Pd2)	High scorers are rebellious and have difficulty accepting standards of behavior that impose responsibilities and interfere with personal gratification. They may be unaware of their angry feelings.
4FD (Pd1)	High scorers reject the family situation and report that it is affectionless, stressful and lacking in emotional support.
4SOA (Pd4A)	High scorers feel isolated, misunderstood and put upon. They lack a viable social support system and tend to blame others for their problems. This scale co-fluctuates with 8SOA which is interpreted similarly. These respondents are also likely to score high on 4FD, making the claim that family members and intimates fail to provide support.
6P (Pa2)	High scorers regard themselves as hypersensitive. They believe that they can be emotionally injured more easily than others and that they heal less quickly.
6N (Pa3)	High scorers claim to be moral and virtuous; for female respondents, virtuousity extends to the sexual area. These respondents appear naive and too trusting. They seem to believe that people in general are benign and honest, which justifies their own moral behavior.
8SOA (Sc1A)	See 4SOA. The two scales co-fluctuate markedly despite minimal item overlap.
8COG (Sc2A)	High scorers on this subscale admit to problems similar to those of the high scorer on 2MD: inability to reason, concentrate and remember. However, they believe that their mental processes are not simply obtunded; they have become threateningly strange. Thus, high scorers on 8COG tend to be more disturbed by their cognitive deficits than high scorers on 2MD. The two scales frequently elevate as a pair.
8CON (Sc2B)	High scorers on this scale announce that they are so emotionally upset that they have lost motivation to behave in a constructive or productive fashion. This is often a consequence of cognitive problems that are reflected in high scores on 2MD and/or 8COG. Tends to co-fluctuate with Work Attitude Scale.
9AMO (Ma1)	High scorers hold to the philosophy that a person is foolish not to take every possible advantage of every situation, usually--but not invariably--short of outright violation of the law. They tend to be somewhat selfish, cynical people who perceive life as an endless series of minor skirmishes in which the person who is not overburdened with scruples is usually victorious. They also believe that most other people share their views.
9PMA (Ma2)	This subscale is a measure of sensation-seeking. High scorers have a high optimal stimulation level, a strong "need for varied, novel, and complex sensations and experience and the willingness to take physical and social risks for the sake of such experience" (Zuckerman, 1979). This subscale is most probably the explanation of why only Scale 9 of the MMPI clinical scales has consistent positive correlations with Zuckerman's Sensation Seeking Scale.
9IMP (Ma3)	See 3DSA.

THE WIGGINS CONTENT SCALES

There have been a number of attempts to create new scales by a factor analysis of the MMPI item pool. None has proven as clinically successful as the effort by Wiggins (1966). The explanation of Wiggins' success probably lies in the unconventionality of his methodology.

Any statistical technique that employs samples is subject to error and that includes factor analysis and similar mathematical techniques. This means that in each factor or cluster, there will be some test items that are erroneously assigned to that factor or cluster.

There are at least two procedures for correcting such erroneous assignments and Wiggins employed both. The first is what might be called "expert judgment as to face validity" or what Wiggins termed "intuitive." Wiggins and a colleague examined each factor, identified items which did not appear to fit logically with the factor to which the original analysis had assigned them, and transferred these items to factors with which their content appeared more congruent.

Wiggins also computed correlation coefficients between each item and each of the total factor scores. Those items which had coefficients below .30 or which had higher correlations with any other factor than the one in which it was included were eliminated.

Wiggins does not give the number of items that were manipulated as a function of clinical judgment although the text suggests that the number was considerable. More than 200 items were eliminated as a function of the content analysis. These methodological maneuvers may very well account for the substantial clinical success of the final scales developed by Wiggins.

Fifteen scales resulted from the procedure described thus far. Two of these lacked sufficient internal consistency even after the removal of items and Wiggins decided to abandon them "on the grounds of unpromising homogeneity." The remaining 13 scales have all proven clinically useful.

It should be considered as a tribute to Wiggins' methodology that two of the most recent factor analyses of the MMPI item pool (Johnson, Null, Butcher, & Johnson, 1984; Foerstner, 1986) emerged with approximately the same factors as did Wiggins more than two decades ago.

Clinical Interpretations of the Wiggins Scales

Interpretations of the Wiggins scales have been proposed by Lachar and Alexander (1978) and Graham (1987) as well as by Wiggins himself (1966). Graham also suggested interpretations for low scores on each of the scales. However, the Wiggins Scales, like most special scales, are unidirectional. Low scores, except for women on the Feminine Interests Scale, have no practical significance.

Table 3.4 presents the interpretations for high scores suggested by Wiggins and Lachar and Alexander. They differ generally in the amount of detail; Lachar and Alexander present a terse summary, Wiggins offers somewhat more detail. Nevertheless, it should be obvious that the two sources are in high agreement concerning interpretation. For each scale, some notes have been added that follow from extended clinical use of these useful scales.

There is a fair number of published reports in the literature using the Wiggins Scales. Only Barron's Ego-Strength Scale and Welsh's A and R Factors appear to have received more attention. By contrast with the latter scales, the reports on the Wiggins Scales are almost unanimously positive, for example, Wiggins, Goldberg,and Applebaum (1971); Taylor, Ptacek, Carithers, Griffin, and Coyne (1972); Payne and Wiggins (1972); Loper, Kammeier, and Hoffmann (1973); Kammeier, Hoffmann, and Loper (1973); Hoffmann, Loper, and Kammeier (1974); Mezzich, Damarin, and Erickson (1974); Boerger (1975); Jarneke and Chambers (1977); Lachar and Alexander (1978); and Woodward, Robinowitz, and Penk (1980). As a group, these investigations provide support for the validity of the Wiggins scales and their appropriate application with a variety of different populations.

TABLE 3.4
Interpretations of the Wiggins' Content Scales

	By Wiggins (1966)	By Lachar & Alexander (1978)	Comments
Social Maladjustment (SOC)	High SOC is socially bashful, shy, embarrassed, reticent, self-conscious, and extremely reserved. Low SOC is gregarious, confident, assertive, and relates quickly and easily to others. He is fun loving, the life of a party, a joiner who experiences no difficulty in speaking before a group. This scale would correspond roughly with the popular concept of "introversion—extraversion."	Endorsed item content reflects a lack of social skill and poise, discomfort in social interaction, and resultant inhibition and social isolation. In client populations this lack of social supports may be associated with a negative self-image, feelings of despair or fearfulness, thoughts of suicide, or a defensive orientation characterized by apathy and limited activity or compulsive attention to detail.	Wiggins' interpretation of low scores on SOC does not mesh with clinical experiences. SOC is a one-tailed scale. Also, suicidal ideation is uncommon in high scorers.
Depression (DEP)	High DEP experiences guilt, regret, worry, unhappiness, and a feeling that life has lost its zest. He experiences difficulty in concentrating and has little motivation to pursue things. His self-esteem is low, and he is anxious and apprehensive about the future. He is sensitive to slight, feels misunderstood, and is convinced that he is unworthy and deserves punishment. In short, he is classically depressed.	This individual has admitted to symptoms associated with problematic depression, such as lack of interest in the environment, pessimism, selfcriticism, and brooding. In client populations social withdrawal, a negative self-concept, guilt feelings, and a reduced activity level may be suggested.	Wiggins states the case well. But some high DEP persons may simply be screaming loudly for help, not "classically" depressed.

	By Wiggins (1966)	By Lachar & Alexander (1978)	Comments
Feminine Interests (FEM)	High FEM admits to liking feminine games, hobbies, and vocations. He denies liking masculine games, hobbies and vocations. Here there is almost complete contamination of content and form that has been noted in other contexts by several writers. Individuals may score high on this scale by presenting themselves as liking many things since this item stem is present in almost all items. They may also score high by endorsing interests, which, although possibly feminine, are also socially desirable, such as an interest in poetry, dramatics, news of the theater, and artistic pursuits. This has been noted in the case of Wiggins' Sd [Social Desirability] scale. Finally, of course, individuals with a genuine preference for activities that are conceived by our culture as "feminine" will achieve high scores on this scale.	Inventory responses suggest an interest in pursuits traditionally labeled as feminine and/or dislike of activities stereotyped as masculine. Patient male: In male clients this interest pattern may be associated with an indecisive, passive orientation that has proven to be problematic. Conflict may lead to confusion or self-blame. Evaluation for suicidal ideation or previous attempts is suggested.	It is risky to draw clinical inferences from high FEM scores in males, especially the better educated. Note that both sources refrain from making inferences about sexual preference. But *very* high scoring females may be protesting too much.

	By Wiggins (1966)	By Lachar & Alexander (1978)	Comments
Poor Morale (MOR)	High MOR is lacking in self-confidence, feels that he has failed in life, and is given to despair and a tendency to give up hope. He is extremely sensitive to the feelings and reactions of others and feels misunderstood by them while at the same time being concerned about offending them. He feels useless and is socially suggestible. There is a substantive overlap here between the Depression and Social Maladjustment scales and the Poor Morale scale. The Social Maladjustment scale seems to emphasize a lack of social ascendance and poise, the Depression scale feelings of guilt and apprehension, while the present scale seems to emphasize a lack of self-confidence and hypersensitivity to the opinions of others.	Inventory responses reflect a pervasive lack of confidence in one's abilities and a history of failure, which is related to these perceived limitations. Clients who obtain high Poor Morale elevations may be insecure, despondent, withdrawn, intropunitive, and oversensitive, and may become easily upset by the actions of others.	MOR is primarily an index of self-image, a measure of self-esteem. Of course, correlations with other depression indicators are expected. MOR also has a correlation of .69 with I-SP, a direct measure of negative self-concept.
Religious Fundamentalism (REL)	High scorers on this scale see themselves as religious, church-going people who accept as true a number of fundamentalist religious convictions. They also tend to view their faith as the true one.	Endorsed item content reflects strong religious beliefs and religiously motivated behavior. In client populations this orientation suggests a reduced probability of substance abuse, impulsive behaviors, and conflict with family members. Expression of strong religious beliefs may, at times, reflect a delusional system and associated thought disorder.	The Lachar–Alexander comments on client groups do not negate Wiggins' interpretation. High REL people may be rigid, dogmatic and intolerant, characteristics that can cause interpersonal conflict.

	By Wiggins (1966)	By Lachar & Alexander (1978)	Comments
Authority Conflict (AUT)	High AUT sees life as a jungle and is convinced that others are unscrupulous, dishonest, hypocritical, and motivated only by personal profit. He distrusts others, has little respect for experts, is competitive, and believes that everyone should get away with whatever they can.	Endorsed item content reflects the belief that interpersonal relations are often exploitive in nature. Disregard for principles of ethical conduct and truthfulness is suggested, as well as a tendency to minimize the negative impact of antisocial behavior. In client populations these attitudes may be associated with problematic overassertive and manipulative social relations. Conflict with relatives may result.	Wiggins' interpretation is extreme. It might apply to respondents who score above T70. For scores in the range T58–69, the Lachar–Alexander interpretation is recommended.
Psychoticism (PSY)	High PSY admits to a number of classic psychotic symptoms of a primarily paranoid nature. He admits to hallucinations, strange experiences, loss of control, and classic paranoid delusions of grandeur and persecution. He admits to feelings of unreality, daydreaming, and a sense that things are wrong, while feeling misunderstood by others.	Inventory responses include admission of unusual experiences and beliefs, many of which may include a clearly paranoid component. In client populations this response pattern often suggests an individual who finds comprehension of human motives and behavior difficult and is consequently suspicious of and worried about others. Symptoms associated with a psychotic adjustment, such as ideas of reference, hallucinations, and autistic or disorganized thought, may be present.	Because of the considerable overlap between PSY and alienation scales, sociopathically inclined individuals who are not psychotic may obtain misleading high scores on PSY.

	By Wiggins (1966)	By Lachar & Alexander (1978)	Comments
Organic Symptoms (ORG)	High ORG admits to symptoms that are often indicative of organic involvement. These include headaches, nausea, dizziness, loss of mobility and coordination, loss of consciousness, poor concentration and memory, speaking and reading difficulty, muscular control, skin sensations, hearing, and smell.	This individual has admitted to a variety of sensory, motor, or general somatic concerns that may be related to psychological discomfort and general malaise as well as to reduced effectiveness in completing daily tasks. Clients who obtain high Organic Symptoms elevations may complain of lack of stamina and strength and may present physical symptoms that often indicate emotional conflict, such as problematic headache or back pain.	ORG symptoms *may* indicate organic involvement or they may reflect a dissociative disorder. The scale itself does not distinguish.
Family Problems (FAM)	High FAM feels that he had an unpleasant home life characterized by a lack of love in the family and parents who were unnecessarily critical, nervous, quarrelsome, and quick tempered. Although some items are ambiguous, most are phrased with reference to the parental home rather than the individual's current home.	Inventory responses include admission of pathology in and among family members. A history of poor relationships with parents is suggested, as well as the absence of positive supports in current family interactions, whether with parents, spouse, or extended family. Patient male: In adult male clients admission of family pathology may reflect not only marital conflict but may also suggest intolerant, overactive individuals and a negative self-concept. Drug abuse and other destructive behavior may be associated.	Lachar–Alexander interpretation of high FAM in client males is not supported by clinical experience. Despite item phrasing, most high FAM scorers are referring to the home in which they currently reside.

	By Wiggins (1966)	By Lachar & Alexander (1978)	Comments
Manifest Hostility (HOS)	High HOS admits to sadistic impulses and a tendency to be cross, grouchy, competitive, argumentative, uncooperative, and retaliatory in his interpersonal relationships. He is often competitive and socially aggressive.	This individual admits to problems in adjustment related to unmodulated expression of anger, resentment of perceived injustices, need for interpersonal dominance, and limited self-control. In client populations the combination of hostility, moodiness, and impulsivity may be associated with assaultive or other antisocial or violent behavior.	HOS is an excellent measure of experienced anger but "sadistic" is a bit extreme.
Phobias (PHO)	High PHO has admitted to a number of fears, many of them of the classically phobic variety such as heights, dark, closed spaces, etc.	This individual admits to a variety of fears and appears to be significantly uncomfortable in many situations. Clients who obtain high PHO elevations are viewed as more anxious, tremulous, worrisome, and phobic than most patients. Depression and social withdrawal may also be indicated.	Almost half of the items in PHO do not refer to phobias directly. Scores as high as T60 may be obtained by individuals who are not phobic.
Hypomania (HYP)	High HYP is characterized by feelings of excitement, well-being, restlessness, and tension.	This individual's self-description suggests a fast personal tempo characterized by enthusiasm, cheerfulness, and perhaps irritability or emotional liability. Clients who obtain high Hypomania elevation are often described as immature, hyperactive, excitable, agitated, and restless. They are unlikely to respond intropunitively to conflict and may manipulate others to reach their goals.	Wiggins' interpretation is valid for scores in the range T60–69. Above T70, the Lachar–Alexander interpretation applies, whether the respondent is a client or not.

	By Wiggins (1966)	By Lachar & Alexander (1978)	Comments
Poor Health (HEA)	High HEA is concerned about his health and has admitted to a variety of gastrointestinal complaints centering around an upset stomach and difficulty in elimination.	A significant number of physical complaints are reflected by item endorsement centering mainly around the digestive system. Individuals who obtain high Poor Health elevations are often considerably worried about their health. Cardiac and pulmonary complaints are also occasionally reported.	

Source: Wiggins (1966) and Lachar & Alexander (1978) (reprinted by permission of the copyright holder, the American Psychological Association, and the authors)

THE TRYON, STEIN, AND CHU CLUSTER SCALES

In the 1960s, Tryon and his associates developed a mathematical method for creating independent scales from a large item pool using a special procedure known as cluster analysis which is similar to the usual factor analytic techniques (Tryon, 1966; Stein, 1968). This esoteric statistical technique was applied to 310 MMPI records representing 220 Veterans Administration Hospital inpatients and outpatients and 90 military officers matched with the patients for age and education. The analysis resulted in seven highly reliable clusters that can be considered to be scales for all practically purposes.

The TSC scales have made only rare appearances in research and little is known about their usefulness from experimental data. Stein (1968) reported means on the seven scales for 20 male samples and 13 female samples, most of which had less than 75 subjects. He also reported intercorrelations with the Omnibus Personality Inventory (Heist & Yonge, 1968), the Edwards Personal Preference Schedule (Edwards, 1959) and the Strong Vocational Interest Blank, an earlier version of the current Strong-Campbell Interest Inventory. The samples were small and select: 50 University of California students studying abroad, 50 forestry students, and 50 "public counseling cases" at the University of California Counseling Center. There was a handful of significant correlation coefficients but their bearing on the validity of the various TSC scales is unclear.

Boerger (1975) obtained TSC scale scores along with 18 other MMPI special scales scores from two samples comprising 679 psychiatric inpatients. Sixty-three criterion variables were employed in a vast fishing expedition similar to the effort by Calvin (1975) previously described. Like Calvin, Boerger used the NOSIE and the GBPRS among his criterion measures.

Boerger analyzed his data by comparing mean scores for the highest scoring 25% of the sample on each scale with the remainder of the sample, and the lowest scoring 25% with the remainder of the sample. A rationale for the use of this weak method of analysis is not offered. A correlational technique would seem to be more appropriate and potentially revealing. Even a comparison of the upper and lower quartiles would make more sense.

A bit less than 15% of all the mean comparisons for the TSC scales were significant at the 10% level—a coincidence that has a suspicious smell of chance. Boerger's criterion however, was significance in both samples; his reasoning was that $.10 \times .10 = .01$. A very much smaller number of comparisons reached Boerger's criterion. Since this was an inpatient group, TSC/S, TSC/D and TSC/A did much better than TSC/I, TSC/B, and TSC/R and there is a suggestion of support for validity for the former threesome. But this consideration applies only to the TSC scales as measures of psychopathology. The Boerger data, at best inconclusive, do not bear on the utility of the TSC scales as personality measures.

TABLE 3.5
Interpretation of the Tryon, Stein and Chu Scales

TSC Scale	Interpretation
Body Symptoms	High scorers are anxious about their physical health; they claim to have a variety of physical symptoms of the type commonly associated with anxiety and depression such as pains, easy fatigability, feelings of weakness and minor gastrointestinal complaints.
Depression	High scorers are depressed, unhappy, brood a great deal, and feel under chronic tension. They lack energy and feel useless, incapable and guilty.
Resentment	High scorers tend to express hostility in a typically adolescent pattern; they tend to feel imposed upon and denigrated and are likely to be impatient and irritable.
Social Introversion	High scorers are shy, socially uncomfortable, easily embarrassed and tend to withdraw when faced by stress, especially in situations involving interpersonal relations.
Suspicion	High scorers are likely to be cynical and opportunistic and to mistrust the sincerity and benigness of the motivations of others. They may have a sociopathic orientation but are not necessarily paranoid in the classical sense. Low scorers tend to be naive and suggestible and are relatively easily manipulated.
Tension	High scorers are anxiety-prone, claim to worry chronically, tend to become tense easily.

Clinically, all the TSC scales except TSC/A have been found to be useful measures. Table 3.5 provides the clinically based interpretations of these six scales.

THE INDIANA RATIONAL SCALES

The continued use of Lushene's program over the years, with several revisions, at the Indiana University Medical Center led to the realization that existing MMPI scales did not successfully tap certain important areas. Psychologists at the Medical Center who were involved with Lushene's program decided to create some new scales covering the uncovered areas. The technique was face validity following from the title of the scale, a rational rather than an empirical process. This method has been demonstrated to be the most effective procedure for selecting items for inventory scales (Ashton & Goldberg, 1973; Jackson, 1975; Gynther, Burkhart, & Hovanitz, 1979).

Seven scales were developed by means of expert judgments. Three judges[4] determined the items for four of the scales. Only those items were included that were agreed upon by all three judges.

Severe Reality Distortions (I-RD) (18 items)
Dissociative Symptoms (I-DS) (8 items)
Obsessive-Compulsiveness (I-OC) (9 items)
Sex Problems (I-SP) (14 items[5])

A fourth judge[6] was added for the creation of two additional scales:

Self-Concept (I-SC) (13 items)
Dependency (I-De) (9 items)

Only those items were included that were agreed upon by three of the four judges. A seventh scale, Dominance (I-Do) (17 items), was developed independently by the author.

Since the judges, as clinical psychologists, shared a common educational background as well as a common workplace, the concepts used as scale titles were not defined. The only instruction was that every scale item should be manifestly face valid, requiring little or no inference to justify its inclusion in the scale. There were two special conditions. It was understood beforehand by the judges that only items dealing directly with hallucinations and delusions should be selected for I-RD. In selecting items for I-De, the judges began with the 54 items in the Navran Dependency Scale (Navran, 1952).

Severe Reality Distortions Scale

Diagnosing a psychosis with the MMPI or any verbal inventory is always risky (see, for example, Affleck & Garfield, 1960). To begin with, the intensity or degree of disturbance reflected in items is not necessarily an accurate indicator. There

---

4   The judges were Frank J. Connolly, Wm. George McAdoo, and the author, who in 1977 formed
     Multiphasic Data Analysis Corporation for the purpose of marketing a computerized MMPI
     scoring system. At that time, the Indiana scales were unofficially known as MDAC scales.

5   Only 12 items are scored for female respondents.

6   The fourth judge was Richard J. Lawlor.

are a number of explanations for high-ranging, psychotic-like clinical profiles on the MMPI. Such profiles are obtained by respondents "faking bad" for whatever reason, severe obsessive–compulsives. and individuals lacking sufficient reading comprehension. Diagnosis by critical items taken individually is also a method with minimal reliability.

As Koss, Butcher, and Hoffman (1976) noted:

> Single items are risky sources of important clinical interpretation compared to scales of multiple items. A patient can misread, misinterpret, or mismark a response to a single item and invalidate the item as a correct sample of behavior. (p. 923)

Evidence comes from a small investigation conducted at Indiana University Hospitals. The MMPI was administered to 20 consecutive patients admitted to the hospital in the summer of 1979. Records were scored for a selected set of 46 critical items of which only 11 overlapped with the F Scale. A total of 181 critical items were endorsed by all patients, a mean of just a bit more than nine per patient. One or 2 days after, each patient was interviewed concerning the critical items. Thirty percent of the endorsements—nearly three per patient on the average—were denied. The patients insisted that they had never endorsed about two out of three of the denied items and had misinterpreted one of three. Fifty-two percent of the items dealing with severe reality distortions, such as hallucinations and delusions, were denied or misinterpreted.

A reasonable conception is that the most reliable method of diagnosing psychosis with the MMPI is by means of a scale that encompasses all items for which an endorsement appears to indicate the existence or recent existence of an hallucination or delusion. There are 18 such items on the MMPI; they constitute I-RD.

Clinical experience indicates that I-RD is, indeed, the most reliable psychotic indicator that can be formed from the MMPI pool. It is superior for this purpose to the six signs proposed by Peterson (1954), the ratio developed by Sines and Silver (1963) or Wiggins' Psychoticism Scale, although the later is a useful measureful of the intensity of emotional disturbance.

Not all high scorers on I-RD are psychotic but the probability of psychosis is sufficiently high so that attention should be called to the possibility in the clinical report.

Dissociative Symptoms Scale

I-DS consists of eight items for which the deviant response clearly suggests the presence of a dissociative symptom. Hysteroid personalities are likely to have elevations of T60; individuals scoring at T70 or above are usually the victims of severe dissociative disorders except when I-RD is also significantly elevated. In such instances, the dissociative symptoms are part of the psychosis complex.

Obsessive–Compulsiveness Scale

I-OC consists of nine statements. Three are obvious compulsive rituals, three describe obsessive rumination and three are indicative of obsessive persistence and caution. Individuals with obsessional traits or even obsessive–compulsive personalities rarely score high on I-OC. A high score on I-OC indicates severe obsessive–compulsive disorder, either as neurosis or as an aspect of a psychotic disorder.

Self-Concept

I-SC measures the extent to which the individual has a negative self-image. Its 14 items contain only three that are found on Scale 2. Individuals scoring high on this scale are low in self- esteem and self-confidence, regard themselves as relatively incapable and generally unattractive.

Sex Problems

I-SP was originally composed of 15 items. Experience with clinical use of this scale indicated that one item should be dropped and that two others should be scored only for male respondents. Accordingly, the current version has 14 items that are scored for the male respondent and 12 for the female respondent.Individuals scoring high on I-SP may have any one of a variety of sexual dysfunctions. The scale is not useful in diagnosing paraphilias or sexual deviations, however.

Dependency

The 10 items in I-De were chosen from the 57 proposed as a dependency measure by Navran (1954). I-De is somewhat lacking in effective psychometric properties, notably the distribution of scores tends to be limited. However, I-De is still useful when interpreted together with the Indiana Dominance Scale (I-Do).

Dominance

The 17 items of this scale describe an individual who has strong views that are strongly defended, regards himself/herself as relatively independent of the views of others, is outspoken and self-confident. Like I-De, scores on I-Do appear to have a restricted range. Nevertheless, this scale can be usefully interpreted in conjunction with I-De.

The following rules have been found to be effective:

- Dependent individuals will have a score on I-De that is at least T50 and a score on I-Do that is below T40. Males conforming to this pattern tend to be more noticeably passive, submissive and easily manipulated than women with the pattern.

- Individuals with a need to dominate others will have a score on I-Do that is at least T50 and a score on I-De that does not reach as high as T40. Such individuals are not necessarily dominant. The scales describe a need; whether the individual is successful in satisfying this need or not is not reflected in the scale scores.

- Individuals whose scores do not fall into one of the two previous patterns can be said to be unremarkable with respect to their dependency and dominance needs.

SOME SPECIAL SPECIAL SCALES

Among the Harris and Lingoes subscales, the Wiggins Content Scales, the Tryon, Stein, and Chu Cluster Scales and Indiana Scales, there are some 43 clinically proven measures covering a wide range of symptoms and traits. This group of scales substantially exceeds the diagnostic capacity of the conventional clinical scales. But there are a number of other scales of proven utility that should be included in the armamentarium of the clinician who makes use of special scales.

The Pepper and Strong Altruism Scale (5C)

In an unpublished report, Pepper and Strong (1958) proposed a five subscale breakdown of the MMPI Scale 5 (Masculinity– Femininity). The Pepper and Strong breakdown of Scale 5 resulted in the following subscales:

Denial of Masculine Occupational Interest (5DMO)
Feminine Occupational Interests (5FO1)

Personal and Emotional Sensitivity (5PES)
Sexual Identification (5SI)
Altruism (5A)

The Pepper and Strong scales are probably superior to the breakdown of Scale 5 suggested by Serkownek (Schuerger, Foerstner, Serkownek, & Ritz, 1987). However, clinical experience indicates that only one of the Pepper and Strong scales is independently useful.

5DMO and 5FOI are neatly encompassed in Wiggins Feminine Interests Scale. 5PES is redundant with the Harris and Lingoes Poignancy Scale (6P). 5SI is mislabeled and is not useful.

Individuals scoring high on 5A endorse traditional American cultural values like honesty, candor, and fair play. They tend to be somewhat unsophisticated; scale scores have moderate positive correlations with 3NA and 6AMV and are also positively related to Lie Scale scores. "Altruism" hardly seems to be a good descriptor for this scale although no doubt high scorers would agree that generosity and selflessness are virtues. *Conventionality* appears to be a more appropriate label, thus 5C.

Cynicism Scale (E/Cy)

One of the several factor analyses of the MMPI pool was carried out by Eichman, originally with female inpatients (Eichman, 1961) and later extended to male inpatients (Eichman, 1962). In both investigations, four factors were identified. The first three were labeled Anxiety, Repression, and Somatization. Eichman was uncertain about the label for Factor IV. At first, he decided to call it Acting-Out on the grounds that the clinical loadings suggested that the factor might be measuring either psychoticism or sociopathy. After collecting the male data, Eichman decided to call Factor IV Unconventionality on the grounds that the item content "carries the flavor of unconventional, impulsive, and perhaps bizarre behavior..." (p.367). He allowed, however, that "the meaning of a high IV score in the normal population is important but remains to be done" (p.380).

Factor IV contains 20 items in the scale for males and 20 for females with 14 items in common. Examination of the item content certainly would not lead to an inference that the appropriate title for the scale is Unconventionality. A high scorer on Factor IV would be no more likely to be unconventional than a high scorer on any number of other sets of 20 MMPI items. The content examination suggests that a majority of the items for both males and females appear to be tapping a characteristic that might best be labeled *cynicism*. Most of the remaining items, though they do not appear to be measuring cynicism directly, are at least not sharply incompatible with this assessment.

E/Cy tends to elevate along with alienation and suspicion scales, as in the records of sociopathically inclined individuals, much as might be expected (see Chapter 5). It has minimal or no item overlap with scales measuring alienation and suspicion and thus is a distinct contribution to the measurement of personality tendencies.

The Cook and Medley Hostility Scale (Ho)

Ho was originally part of a group of 77 items chosen because they discriminated between school teachers scoring high and low on the Minnesota Teacher Attitude Inventory. Five clinical psychologists then selected the final 50-item version of Ho on the basis of "substantial agreement" which is not defined by Cook and Medley (1954).

Ho is one of the few special scales that has been used in published research and it has given rise to some interesting findings. Jurjevich (1963) found that Ho did a better job of relating to the subscales of the Buss–Durkee Hostility–Guilt Index (Buss & Durkee, 1957) than five other item sets derived from the MMPI including Scales 4 and 6. McGee (1954) found that Ho had low but significant correlations with a word association test and a picture sorting test designed to measure hostility. Shaw and Grubb (1958) reported that underachieving male high school sophomores obtained a higher Ho score than achievers, according to hypothesis. Ho also correlated .79 for females and .85 for males with the Hostility Scale of the Guilford–Zimmerman Temperament Survey. However, Megargee and Mendelsohn (1962) reported that Ho, like 11 other MMPI measures related to hostility, failed to discriminate among three groups classified as extremely assaultive criminals, moderately assaultive criminals and nonassaultive criminals, and a group of noncriminals.

More recently, Ho has entered the health psychology field. Williams et al. (1980) found a significant relationship between scores on Ho and the severity of coronary artery disease in a sample of more than 400 patients who underwent coronary angiography. In fact, Ho scores predicted the severity more efficiently than interview-based ratings of Type A behavior. Smith and Frohm (1985), in a questionnaire study, reported that high Ho scorers were beset by the combination of a less satisfactory social support system and more frequent irritating events making for what the authors characterize as "a distinctly negative psychosocial risk factor profile" (p.514).

Barefoot, Dahlstrom, and Williams (1983) and Shekelle, Gale, Ostfeld, and Paul (1983) reported that Ho was a predictor of the incidence of heart attacks and cardiac deaths over extended periods of time.

Spielberger, Jacobs, Russell, and Crane (1983) found a significant correlation that averaged around .50 between Ho and the trait form of the State-Trait Anger Scale. A significant correlation was also reported between Ho and estimated potential for hostility based on interviews by Dembroski, MacDougall, Williams, and Haney (1985).

On the whole, the various field studies of Ho are strong testimony to its validity but do not necessarily support the Cook and Medley choice of a scale designation. There is no firm, independently verified theoretical structure from which one could predict that high school underachievers would be more hostile than achievers or that individuals developing coronary artery disease are more given to trait hostility than those who do not.

A recent factor analysis of the MMPI item pool (Johnson, Null, Butcher, & Johnson 1984) resulted in a set of factors that included a 20-item factor labeled by expert decision, Cynicism. Sixteen of those 20 items are common to Ho. Another recent factor analysis of the MMPI pool (Costa, Zonderman, McCrae, & Williams 1985) also resulted in a Cynicism factor with 22 items in common with Ho.

The cynicism content of Ho is so marked that Smith and Frohm (1985) suggest that the scale should be called Cynical Hostility. Their statement of high scores on Ho dovetails neatly with clinical experience:

> High Ho scorers are prone to anger and are suspicious and resentful of others. Though not necessarily more likely to report physical aggressiveness, they view others with distrust and are likely to be vigilant, calculating, and manipulative in their social interactions...These persons are likely to become dysphoric, to feel isolated and dissatisfied with their social supports, and to experience more frequent and subjectively severe daily irritants. (p.516)

Overcontrolled Hostility Scale (OH)

Several reasonably careful investigations arrived at the interesting conclusion that institutionalized criminals convicted of violent crimes tend to score lower on measures of aggression and higher on measures of control than do nonassaultive criminals and normal men (Megargee & Mendelsohn, 1962; Blackburn, 1968). This curious finding led Megargee (1966) to the conclusion that assaultive criminals come in two types: undercontrolled and overcontrolled. Accordingly, he set about devising a scale for the measurement of hostility in the overcontrolled person (Megargee, Cook, & Mendelsohn, 1967).

The 31 items of the OH scale are based on MMPI records of four groups: extremely assaultive men convicted of murder, assault with a deadly weapon, and so on; moderately assaultive men convicted of no more than battery; criminals convicted for crimes other than violence, and normal men. Item analyses resulted in a 55 item scale that differentiated the assaultive from non-assaultive prisoners. However, there was considerable overlap between the distributions. The scale was refined by cross-validation on a new sample of incarcerated offenders. The result was a 31-item scale that not only discriminated assaultive from nonassaultive prisoners but also distinguished between a group of violent criminals classified as overcontrolled and undercontrolled through expert clinical judgment on the basis of examination of prison records.

Megargee et al. (1967) assert that the scale measures simultaneously "two personality contructs which are not normally found together, impulse control and hostile alienation." Thus, they believe that high scorers on OH have serious conflict between strong aggressive impulses and perhaps stronger inhibitions against the expression of aggression. The net consequence is that the hostile impulses are chronically restrained until they mount to a critical intensity at which point the individual is likely to explode into a sudden act of extreme violence or perhaps psychosis.

The OH scale is one of the few that has been subjected to a considerable amount of postdevelopment investigation. Most of the reported investigations support the validity of OH in one way or another (deGroat & Adamson, 1973; Blackburn, 1972; Fredericksen, 1975; Haven, 1972; Lane & Kling, 1979; Megargee, 1969; Vanderbeck, 1973; White, 1970, 1975; White, McAdoo, & Megargee, 1973). Those investigations in which positive findings for validity were not obtained used unsound methodology: administering OH in isolation instead of within the entire MMPI (Lester, Perdue, Brookhart, 1974; Mallory & Walker, 1972; Rawlings, 1973) or using criterion groups that were contaminated by racial bias (Fisher, 1970).

OH was developed with male prisoners and almost all of the subsequent work has tested male samples. The single investigation which included female murderers reported some evidence that OH could also apply to women (Sutker and Allain, 1979). However, the evidence for validity is not strong and this is one of the few studies that did not support the ability of OH to discriminate among male prisoners.

The clinical utility of OH would be very restricted if it were applicable only to samples of incarcerated criminals. As it happens, the value of this interesting set of items ranges considerably beyond such limitations. Clinically, we find that noncriminal male and female high scorers on OH behave very much in accordance with the theoretical position of Megargee et al. (1967). They appear to have strong inhibitions against the expression of aggression and characteristically deny hostile feelings, usually obtaining low scores on such scales as HOS. They are considered to be quiet, passive, and unassuming. They are also given to aperiodic rage reactions in which they may or may not attack others or destroy property. They are rarely murderers.

Table 3.6 provides MMPI data on a single, white, unemployed male, age 34 with an eighth-grade education. He was referred by the police after 20 arrests for public intoxication which often included violent behavior.

Scores on manifest hostility (AUT and HOS) were quite low. The respondent's score on the TSC Resentment scale is within limits. His OH score is

Table 3.6

A Case Illustrating the Use of Special Scales to Identify Overcontrolled Hostility*

AUT	HOS	TSC/R	OH	AMac
39	39	49	73	26

*The AMac datum is a raw score; all others are T-scores.

The patient is male, white, single, age 34, unemployed.

very high and his AMac indicates that he is probably an alcoholic (see Chapter 4 for a discussion of AMac).

An appropriate interpretation would be that this individual typically represses hostility, that he is able to obtain release from the emotional strain of denial and repression by becoming disinhibited with alcohol at which times he acts out aggressively.

Assertiveness

Occasionally, a special scale constructor using the contrasting groups technique will fail in the designed purpose but will succeed serendipitously in creating a new useful scale. The unsuccessful aim of an investigation by Ohlson and Wilson (1974) was to distinguish homosexual from heterosexual females using an inventory composed of MMPI items. The contrasting groups were a sample of lesbians who were active in the gay liberation movement and a carefully matched sample of heterosexual females.

All raw score differences between the two groups on the clinical scales and the conventional validity scales were small although the heterosexual group scored significantly higher on Scales 1, 3, and 7. Fifty-six items differentiated the two groups at the 2% level or beyond; of course, two of these were items No. 69 "I am strongly attracted to members of my own sex," and No. 430 "I am attracted by members of the opposite sex."

Unfortunately, Ohlson and Wilson do not give mean scores on the 56 items for their contrasting groups but clinical experience suggests that while the lesbian group doubtlessly scored higher than the heterosexual sample, there was considerable overlap of the distributions. Using the items diagnostically would result in a spate of false positives. The 56 items as a scale are not recommended for identifying homosexual females.

Examination of the content of the items suggests that they tap not lesbianism but a correlative characteristic of members of the gay liberation movement—assertiveness. Assertiveness is used in this sense as a non-noxious behavior apart from aggression (e.g., Hollandsworth, 1977; Hollandsworth & Wall, 1977). Twenty percent of the items deal directly with this characteristic; most of these were referred to as representing a "masculine orientation" by Ohlson and Wilson. Another large group of items deal with physical health and emotional adjustment which are not unreasonable associated with assertiveness in women. About 10% of the items are stereotypically feminine characteristics that are likely not to be found in assertive women.

Clinical experience suggest that an Assertiveness scale (Astvn) for women composed of the Ohlson–Wilson items except for Nos. 69 and 430, has assessment value.

THE OBVIOUS–SUBTLE DISTINCTION
APPLIED TO SPECIAL SCALES

As has already been pointed out, an early demonstration of the multidimensionality of MMPI clinical scales was the separation of items into obvious and subtle categories. In principle, an obvious item is one for which the significance of a true or false response should be manifest to most respondents. Few adults would have difficulty comprehending the meaning of endorsement of items like "I work under a great deal of tension," or "I have had very peculiar and strange experiences." On the other hand, the assessment meaning of endorsing an item like "At times I feel that I can make up my mind with unusually great ease," or denying "I like to talk about sex" would not be understood by most respondents.

Wiener and Harmon

The original classification of MMPI items as obvious or subtle was the work of Wiener and Harmon (1946), later published under Wiener's name (Wiener, 1948, 1956). Wiener and Harmon essentially used two methods of distinguishing items. All items on the F Scale and on Scales 1, 7, 8 were automatically assigned to the obvious category on the grounds that they measured psychopathology, presumably directly, although this is not specifically stated. Most of the remaining items were categorized by the authors' "pooled judgments"; the procedure is not detailed any further.

It is plain that by "obvious" Wiener and Harmon meant that the item clearly described a bit of psychopathology on a particular clinical scale. This point is indicated by the fact that there are eight items keyed in the same direction that were designated as obvious on one scale and subtle on another. For example, the item "My hardest battles are with myself" (True) is classified as obvious on Scale 7 and subtle on Scale 4.

The notion that an item can be obvious on one scale and subtle on another is not sensible. It hints at the ridiculous possiblity that respondents not only can determine the significance of endorsement or denial of the item but can also determine to which clinical scale or scales the item belongs. It makes more sense simply to judge whether or not the average respondent could tell whether or not a response admits to psychopathology.

Weiner (1948, 1956) reported early that the obvious sets of items were not statistically related to the subtle items. The average intercorrelation was -.50. The highest positive correlation was only .24 (Scale 9). He also reported that the obvious items alone differentiated successful from unsuccessful students and job trainees while the total scores on the clinical scales did not differentiate.

These two findings have been reported from a number of sources over the years, most recently by Wrobel and Lachar (1982). The incapacity of the subtle items of the MMPI is a telling argument against the use of the clinical scales and in favor of a battery of special scales.

Another Approach to the Obvious–Subtle Distinction

All that we know about psychological measurement suggests that the approach to the obvious–subtle distinction used by Weiner and Harmon is too simplistic. Few phenomena of human life are naturally dichotomous; there should be degrees of obviousness and subtlety. Indeed, this seems to be the case. One could easily dispute the assignment of an item like "My hands and feet are usually warm enough," or "I loved my father" to the obvious category, or "At times I have very much wanted to leave home," or "My hardest battles are with myself" to the subtle category. These items, like many others, appear to be not quite obvious and not quite subtle.

Christian, Burkhart, and Gynther (1978) approached the obvious–subtle distinction from the position that obvious and subtle are ends of a dimension rather than merely a dichotomy. They asked a large group of college students to make estimates on a 5-point scale ranging from 1 (most subtle) to 5 (most obvious). The mean estimate per item was then computed. In this procedure, "I have a good appetite," has a mean rating of 2.91 and "My hands and feet are usually warm

TABLE 3.7
A Comparison of Subtlety on the MMPI Clinical Scales

Scale		Percent Subtle Items	
		Wiener & Harmon	Christian et al.*
F		0	6
Hs	(1)	0	9
D	(2)	33	30
Hy	(3)	47	37
Pd	(4)	43	22
Pa	(6)	43	23
Pt	(7)	0	2
Sc	(8)	0	1
Ma	(9)	50	35
Overall		23	17.7

*Items having a mean rating of 2.5 or less.

enough," has a mean rating of 2.67, both on the subtle side of the scale. On the other side of the Weiner and Harmon ledger, "At times I have very much wanted to leave home," received a mean rating of 3.46 and "At times I feel like picking a fist fight with someone," obtained a mean rating of 3.74. Both are at the obvious end of the scale.

The reference group used by Christian et al. is perhaps not the most appropriate one but it does represent a population of potential subjects for the application of the MMPI. More importantly, it provides a more refined statement of obviousness and subtlety than a dichotomous system.

Table 3.7 gives a comparison of the proportions of subtle items assigned to the F Scale and the eight clinical scales compared with the proportions of items that had mean ratings below 2.5, the midpoint of the 5-point scale according to the raters employed by Christian et al.

In general, Wiener and Harmon found more subtle items than did the raters of Christian et al., 23% against 17.7%. Wiener and Harmon made no judgments for the F Scale and for Scales 1, 7, and 8, deciding that all items in those scales were obvious. Computing only for the remaining five scales, the mean subtle percent by Wiener and Harmon is 57, by Christian et al. only 30. Nevertheless, it appears that Wiener and Harmon were not far afield when they decided to deal only with five scales. The mean subtle percentage for Scales 1, 7, and 8 and the F Scale according to the raters of Christian et al. is only 4.5.

The difference in assignments between Wiener and Harmon and the Christian et al. raters may be partly a function of improved diagnostic skills over a 30-year period. It is also clearly due to the effect of the 5-point as opposed to the 2-point categorization. Wiener and Harmon apparently assigned more of the doubtful items to the subtle category, for whatever reasons.

Using the Obvious–Subtle Ratings. Obvious–subtle ratings based on the work of Christian et al. were computed for each special scale described in this volume by averaging the ratings of its items. These means are presented along with their respective scales in Appendix IV.

The common practice among high-point code typologists is to discard the faking bad record as invalid and therefore uninterpretable. Even when the respondent is indeed faking bad, there will be some scales among the special scales that may still be validly interpreted. Exaggeration of psychopathology is almost always accomplished by endorsements of obvious items. The point appears uncontestable; how could a respondent fake if he/she was unable to fathom the significance of a true or false response to the item? The empirical demonstration of this axiom by Burkhart, Christian, and Gynther (1978) is almost gratuitous.

In general, scales that have a definite obvious quality such as PSY whose mean rating is 3.86 or 8COG with 3.74 would be risky to interpret in a record with elevated Cl, TR, and/or ME. On the other hand, AMac (O–S rating = 2.63), OH (2.39), and 3DSA (2.10) can be interpreted with reasonably safety even in the faking bad record. In general, a scale with a mean item rating of less than 3.00 will be interpretable.

CHAPTER 4
THE ASSESSMENT
OF PSYCHOPATHOLOGY

There is still debate about whether the MMPI was originally intended to assess personality but there is little doubt that a primary purpose was to assist in diagnosing psychopathology. The titles of the original clinical scales testified to this aim with abundant clarity. Hathaway and McKinley (1951, p.6) stated flatly that "a high score on a scale has been found to predict positively the corresponding final clinical diagnosis or estimate in more than 60 per cent of new psychiatric admissions."

This optimistic prediction was never verified. In fact, it rapidly became clear that many psychiatric patients, especially those who were seriously disturbed, would be more likely to have two elevated clinical scales rather than a lone "spike." The concept of the 2-point code type was in place early on (Hathaway, 1947) and within a decade, was to become the orthodoxy. The official policy now was that assigning numbers to the scales was an attempt to escape from the misleading diagnostic connotations of the original scale labels. It was formally acknowledged that "it had become apparent with widespread testing that many people who scored high on the Sc scale were by no means clinically schizophrenic" (Welsh & Dahlstrom, 1956, p.124). Coding now was advanced as "a positive approach to the clinical and research problems with the MMPI" (Welsh & Dahlstrom, 1956, p.124).

The same "widespread testing" also demonstrated that code typology was not much more successful as a diagnostic tactic than the use of single scales. The next step was the development of rules based on all or most of the clinical scales such as those devised by Meehl and Dahlstrom (1960) and Goldberg (1965). These systems were designed not to make specific diagnoses but simply to distinguish among broad categories of diagnostic entities such as psychosis and neurosis.

A recent summary and extension of investigations of these diagnostic methods shows that they, too, have failed (Pancoast, Archer, & Gordon, 1988). The accuracy of diagnostic identification by several systems ranged from about one quarter to one third of cases examined, not very far from chance expectation and too weak to be of value to the practicing clinician.

THE MEASUREMENT OF SYMPTOMS

With the exception of the five-scale system created by Rosen (1962), special scales have not been devised for differential diagnosis and there has been no suggestion that they should be employed in this manner. Various special scales are intended to measure symptoms and personality characteristics. Mental health treatment is more often linked to specific symptoms rather than to diagnostic entities so this is no deficiency in the special scales. However, while there are a number of special scales that are intended to assess symptoms of all sorts, only a few of them have been tested, either experimentally or clinically. The capacities of those that have been examined clinically vary, but all share a common defect that is inherent in the MMPI item pool. Because of the phrasing of most symptom items, symptom-measuring special scales appear to be trait measures. Experience indicates that these scales also reflect states in the usual sense that trait and state are invariably positively correlated. At the moment of measurement in the individual case, the clinician must decide on the basis of other evidence whether the special scale is measuring state as well as trait.

Anxiety

No MMPI clinical scale is designed to measure anxiety although the role is often assigned to Scale 7. There are a number of special scales specifically created for this purpose. Unfortunately, clinical experience has not included all of them. The two best-known special scales intended to measure anxiety, Taylor's Manifest Anxiety Scale (MAS; Taylor, 1953) and Welsh's A Factor (Welsh, 1956) have not proven clinically useful. The primary reason in the case of the MAS is that it is heavily loaded with physical symptom items—13 of its 50. It has a marked tendency to elevate when the respondent is prone to somatize but does not have anxiety, worry, apprehension, and the like, as a primary symptom, except, perhaps, where their physical symptoms are concerned. The A Scale, in the light of today, appears to be a yea-saying measure of a tendency to psychological maladjustment that includes items that tap symptoms other than anxiety such as depression, guilt, hypersensitivity, and obsessive–compulsiveness. In fact, it appears that there are more depression items on the A Scale than items that measure anxiety directly.

Clinical usage suggests that the two most effective measures of anxiety among special scales are the Tryon, Stein, and Chu Tension Scale (TSC/T) and the Wiggins Phobia Scale (PHO). The former is a measure of *anxiety-proneness* or *free-floating anxiety* or *general apprehension*—whatever term connotes to the reader that the anxiety measured tends to be relatively vague and diffuse. By comparison, of course, a phobia should be a compartmentalized, sharply defined, specific fear. Unfortunately, it is by no means a simple matter to determine when a fear should be called a phobia (the reader is referred to the discussion on this point in Levitt, 1980, pp. 6-8). Actually, it appears that no more than 15 of the 27 items in PHO qualify as phobias. But because the expected means on PHO are about 7 for men and about 10 for women, it would be most unusual to have a significant elevation on PHO without endorsement of a number of phobia items.

There is an overlap of 11 items between PHO and TSC/T. Of these 11 items, 4 are clearly not phobias, 3 are phobias and 4 others are questionable.

Item overlap, which amounts to 31% for TSC/T and 41% for PHO, unquestionably accounts partly for the correlation of .71 between the scales for both males and females. Obviously, we expect these two scales to cofluctuate, not only because of the item overlap but for sound theoretical reasons. Most people who are anxiety-prone have specific fears. However, the employment of both scales is still useful since individuals who score high on one and low on the other are not rare. Some anxiety-prone individuals are general worriers and tend not to bind anxiety in specific fears. At the other end of the spectrum, some individuals do such an effective job of binding free-floating anxiety that they appear only as phobic.

Depression

Depression, the most common diagnosis and symptom in the mental health field, is a vast, complex, labyrinthine monster (Levitt, Lubin, & Brooks, 1983). The term is used variably as the designation of a mood state, a symptom, syndrome, as well as a diagnostic entity. Theoreticians have suggested that not everyone who is depressed is manifestly unhappy and certainly not everyone who is unhappy is depressed. Surely depressed people occasionally take their own lives but what are the markers that determine that a depressed person requires hospitalization and/or antidepressant medication?

The problem with MMPI Scale 2 (Depression) is that it bears a heavy load of items dealing with physical health. There are 13 such items, more than 20% of the total. In their breakdown of Scale 2, Harris and Lingoes (1955) assigned 11 of those items to the Physical Malfunctioning subscale (2PM). The removal of those items would make Scale 2 a more realistic measure of subjective depression.

No one would deny that depressed people are beset by health problems. On the contrary, there is a frequent association between the subjective feeling of depression and bodily symptoms. However, there are other scales available for the measurement of health concerns.

Physical symptom items are not included either in Wiggins' DEP, which has 33 items nor in TSC/D, which has 28. Thus, both of these are superior measures of the affective and cognitive aspects of depression.

DEP and TSC/D have a not surprising overlap of 14 items and an intercorrelation for both men and women of .94. Obviously, the two scales cofluctuate tightly with each other. In addition, they also have correlations ranging from .80 to .90 with Harris and Lingoes subscales 2SD (Subjective Depression) and 2MD (Mental Dullness). The correlations with 2PM range only from .39 to .43, which is a statistical illustration of the value of using depression scales that are not weighted with bodily symptom items.

Suicide Potential. One of the most significant assessments that is made by mental health professionals is the probability that a patient will commit suicide. The suicide rate among individuals diagnosed as depressives, schizophrenics, and alcoholics is significantly greater than the rate in the general population (Levitt, Lubin, & Brooks, 1983). A not infrequent rationale for hospitalization is that the individual appears to pose the threat of suicide. Thus, accurate prediction is extremely important and it is not surprising to find that a fair number of studies have been devoted to attempts to assess suicide potential using MMPI scales or items. Clopton (1979b) authored the most recent review of this literature.

Two inferences may be drawn from Clopton's review: (a) The clinical scales have been unsuccessful in predicting suicide potential; and (b) At least four suicide potential scales have independently developed from the MMPI item pool. None of these appears to be a successful measure of suicide potential.

Apparently, no one has tried to use already existing MMPI special scales to assess suicide potential. A popular hypothesis concerning the relationship between depression and suicide suggests that certain special scales may indeed be effective in predicting the suicide possibility.

This view holds that the depressed person contains within his/her symptomatology an essence that militates against self-destruction, namely, that the sufferer lacks the energy and drive to do away with him or herself. Improvement in the depressive symptoms may *increase* the suicide risk, a not uncommon clinical observation (for example, Pokorny, 1968; Klerman, 1982). As Pokorny (1968) pointed out, "the greatest risk of suicide is during the period of improvement; at this time the patient may regain sufficient drive or energy to take his life" (p. 71). It might be inferred that it is not only after improvement has taken place that risk heightens but at any time when the patient is badly disturbed but *not severely apathetic or anergic.*

The Psychomotor Retardation subscale of Scale 2 (2PR) contains the subset of depression items that tap apathy and anergy. The Subjective Depression subscale of Scale 2 (2SD) contains the depression items that deal with subjective feelings of unhappiness, guilt, worthlessness, and so on. [1] The correlation between 2PR and 2SD is only .38 for males, .56 for females, and .48 for the total sample. Some part of this relationship is surely due to an interscale overlap of eight items. Evidently, at least some individuals with high scores on 2SD are likely to have low scores on 2PR. This differential occurs among psychiatric patients as well as in normative groups.

Among depressed patients, those with the expected high scores on 2SD but with low scores on 2PR would logically be the suicide risks. Unfortunately, there has been no objective investigation of the possible predictive capacity of the 2PR-2SD combination. Clinical experience is scanty but there has been at least a few cases in which a score of T70 or higher on 2SD with a score of less than T60 on 2PR was associated with a suicide attempt. It is a worthwhile possibility to be checked out by the MMPI clinician.

Chronic Low-Grade Depression. Although many of the special scales that measure personality factors are unidirectional, most symptom scales are not. A high score on PHO suggests that the respondent is beset by phobias. A low score is interpreted to mean that the respondent is free from phobic symptoms.

This reasoning applies also to depression, but not quite. True, a high score on DEP or TSC/D suggests that the individual is depressed and a low score that he/she is not depressed. "Not depressed" in the clinical sense yet not necessarily happy or content with his/her life space. Some people have minimal feelings of being in a "down" mood, have no outstanding guilt feelings, nor cognitive symptoms of depression. Yet, they find living to be a trial. Matters do not necessarily go wrong for them; they just don't seem to go right. Such individuals seldom feel elated or attain a truly "up" mood and tend to be a bit cross and irritable more often than persons who do not have this chronic low-grade depression. Should they encounter a mental health professional, they would probably be diagnosed as Schizoid Personality Disorder or perhaps Depressive State NOS. Most avoid that encounter although they find their way frequently to the nonpsychiatric medical practitioner.

Chronic low-grade depressives tend to score within normal limits on DEP, TSC/D, and 2SD though often in the range T55 and occasionally above T60 on one of these scales. The critical scale elevation for this diagnosis is the Wiener and Harmon Depression-Subtle set of items (see Chapter 3). An elevation of at least T60 on D-S when the depression scales do not reach that level is the mark of the chronically discontented individual.

---

1   Notably, 4 of the 15 items in 2PR and 10 of the 32 items in 2SD--30% of the items in the two scales--are included in the 52-item Suicide Threat scale developed by Farberow and Devries (1967).

The Measurement of Psychoticism

Beyond the structural defects of MMPI clinical scales noted in Chapter 1, the identification of psychoticism by means of a verbal inventory is always risky and must be tentative. Response sets, poor reading ability, and the opportunity for misunderstandings and idiosyncratic interpretation of items accumulate to plague the clinician in the identification of thought disorders and other severe psychopathology.

The MMPI clinical scales have been no more successful in the diagnosis of psychotism than might be expected. The F Scale, long heralded as a psychotic measure in its own right, frequently elevates when the respondent is psychotic—and often elevates when the respondent is not. Any respondent with a significant elevation on Scale 8, either alone as a spike or in conjunction with Scales 6 and 7, is commonly considered to be schizophrenic. However, there is no doubt whatsoever that a substantial number of people who show elevations on Scale 8 are not psychotic.

There are several other methods of combining clinical scale scores in order to attempt to measure psychoticism, such as Peterson's (1954) six diagnostic signs and Goldberg's (1965) index. None of these attempts has proven sufficiently successful to warrant their common use in clinical facilities.

Obviously, special scales are not immune to the problems of the verbal instrument but at least they have the potential to avoid some of the structural defects of the clinical scales. There are six special scales that have potential utility in diagnosing thought disorder.

Indiana Severe Reality Distortions Scale (I-RD)

I-RD is a face valid instrument that is composed simply of the 18 hallucinations and delusions that are in the MMPI item pool. To be sure, these may be misunderstood; indeed the means of between 1 and 2 for both males and females on this scale in themselves suggest misunderstandings. However, a raw score of 5 for women or 6 for men (that is, T70) is unlikely to be due to item misinterpretations and appears to be pathognomic of a psychotic process.

The Indiana Dissociative Symptoms Scale (I-DS)

I-DS is another face valid scale which is composed of the eight items in the MMPI pool that describe dissociative symptoms such as "I have had periods in which I carried on activities without knowing later what I had been doing," or "I often feel as if things are not real." I-DS contains three I-RD items. This necessitates caution since T70 for males on I-DS is only 3 and for females, 4. Thus, in order to be certain that I-DS is contributing to the symptomatology beyond the score obtained on I-RD, the score on I-DS would have to exceed T70.

While symptoms in I-DS are usually classified as dissociative, they are not infrequently found in psychotic persons. Consider, for example, items such as "My soul sometimes leaves my body," and "I have had some very unusual religious experiences."

Wiggins' Psychoticism Scale (PSY)

PSY numbers among its 48 items all 18 in M-RD, and eight items that form the Harris and Lingoes Bizarre Sensory Experiences subscale of Scale 8 (8BSE). These 26 items, a bit more than half of the complement in PSY, may be considered to be legitimate measures of psychoticism. However, PSY also contains nine items that appear either in 4SOA or 8SOA, or in both. Among sociopathic, disillusioned, or otherwise alienated persons, a high score on 4SOA or 8SOA can cause PSY to elevate spuriously. This is especially true because the overlap of PSY items on either alienation scale is almost equal to a standard deviation unit of PSY. Thus, in assessing the significance of PSY, one must examine the two alienation scales. If they are elevated, then there is a good probability that a high score of PSY does not indicated the presence of psychoticism. On the other hand, if 4SOA and 8SOA are within the normal range, then an elevation on PSY could be pathognomic of a psychotic process.

Paranoia. TSC/S assesses distrustfulness across a broad range of psychological adjustments. It measures suspiciousness as a common trait variable in the general population. High scorers are likely to be suspicious, cynical, and opportunistic with status ranging from normal to sociopathic. They are not likely to be delusional or paranoid in the classical sense. Consider, for example, the diagnostic difference between "Someone has it in for me," which is like the sociopathic externalization of blame and the "Someone is trying to poison me" of the paranoid schizophrenic.

Several special scales are sensitive to paranoid ideation in the respondent, for example, PSY, 6PI, and 8COG. None of these is sufficiently specific. Perhaps one third of the 17 items of 6PI tap paranoia directly, fewer on PSY and 8COG.

A diagnosis involving paranoid ideation is made with reasonable confidence based on a high score on the Extreme Suspiciousness Scale (S+; Endicott, Jortner, & Abramoff, 1969). About half of the 18 items on S+ are clearly paranoid delusions. The remaining items express the hypersensitivity and hypercaution that are like to underly paranoid tendencies. High scorers on S+ are paranoid persons at some level. Not all are psychotic; some will be diagnosed as paranoid personalities or delusional disorders.

The Measurement of Sociopathic Tendency

The behaviors of the antisocial personality disorder as they are described in DSM-III-R (APA, 1987), are essentially those of a criminal and/or vagrant: lying, cheating, pursuing an illegal occupation, failing to plan ahead, wandering without good purpose from place to place, unable to sustain any socially productive or responsible behavior, and generally not following social norms. This pattern is seen in an estimated 3% of the adult population, mostly males, according to DSM-III-R.

There are others who manifest tendencies like the antisocial personality but not necessarily to a psychopathology extreme. Many are not criminals or vagrants and do not warrant a diagnosis of antisocial personality disorder. Even the term *antisocial* appears somewhat amiss when applied to such individuals. The original DSM term *sociopathic* (APA, 1952) seems to describe them more clearly.

These individuals have personality structures that resemble the antisocial personality disorder. They are apt to feel misunderstood and put upon, to externalize blame, to be rebellious, cynical, and suspicious of the motivations of others. Most have never been able to build an effective social support system and usually feel isolated, alone, and perhaps different. Guilt is rarely a prominent feature but hostility and/or depresssion may be manifested. Yet, a large number of individuals with sociopathic tendencies manage to function without intervention and without attracting the attention of authorities of any kind.

Items tapping sociopathic tendencies will be found on Scale 4 and 6 of the MMPI but typically, indistinguishable in a melange of items measuring other characteristics. Certainly, sociopathically inclined persons may elevate on Scale 4 but as we saw in Chapter 1, high scores on this scale may also be obtained by individuals without particular tendency toward sociopathy.

There are 10 special scales that are involved in the identification of the respondent with sociopathic inclinations. Four are Harris and Lingoes subscales: 4AC, 4SOA, 8SOA, and 9AMO. Two are in the Wiggins group: AUT and HOS: two are Tryon, Stein, and Chu scales: TSC/R and TSC/S. The complement is completed by the Cook and Medley (1954) Ho scale and Eichman's (1961) Cynicism Scale (E/Cy).

Alienation. The cornerstone scales in this group are 4SOA and 8SOA which generally cofluctuate despite the fact that they have only four items—approximately 20% of each scale—in common. High scorers on these scales typically feel isolated and lack an effective support system. They also feel generally misunderstood and tend to externalize blame for their problems. Individuals who score above T70 on either scale have a strong sense of being estranged from society and feel discriminated against as well as misunderstood.

These individuals also often score high on the two scales that assess family difficulties: the Harris and Lingoes Familial Discord subscale (4FD) and Wiggins' Family Problems Scale (FAM). Incidentally, the family difficulties scales cofluctuate markedly due to an overlap of eight items which amounts to 50% of the items in FAM and more than 70% of the ones in 4FD.

Cynicism. Frequent accompaniments of alienation are cynicism and suspicion. E/Cy is a relatively pure measure of cynicism, whereas Ho, as indicated in an earlier discussion, taps an amalgam of cynicism and hostility. The overlap between the two scales amounts to 14% for Ho and 27% for E/Cy.

Harris and Lingoes 9AMO tends to elevate with all of the scales mentioned so far, especially the measures of cynicism. Individuals scoring high on 9AMO tend to perceive others as behaving dishonestly, selfishly, and opportunistically and therefore feel justified in behaving similarly. It reflects a kind of a jungle philosophy in which one either takes advantage of others or is taken advantage of by others.

Anger. The best measure of experienced hostility is Wiggins HOS. Individuals who elevate on this scale are aware of their hostility although they may not be aware that it is manifested as often as it actually is. The Tryon, Stein, and Chu Resentment Scale (TSC/R) is also a measure of hostility but of a somewhat different tenor. The anger of people who score high on TSC/R has a pettish, irritable quality, much like an adolescent who reacts negatively to the impression that he/she is being put upon, manipulated, and overpowered by his/her parents. Indeed, adolescents are more likely to elevate on TSC/R than are adults.

Authority Conflict. The two measures of authority conflict—AUT and 4AC—have only three items in common and appear to tap somewhat different aspects of this phenomenon. The correlation between the two scales is only .38 for females and .41 for males and indeed, clinically one sees a substantial number of instances in which 4AC is significantly elevated and AUT is not. Such individuals are unaware of their rebellious inclinations, unlike high scorers on AUT who seem to be aware. Significantly, the correlation between AUT and HOS is .66 for females and .64 for males while the correlation between 4AC and HOS is only .26 and .23.

Suspiciousness. TSC/S measures suspiciousness as a nonpsychotic tendency. Individuals who score in the range T55-T65 on TSC/S tend to be hypercautious and controlled in their interpersonal dealings. Those who score above T65 must be considered to be suspicious people who often question the motives and intentions of others and tend to be doubtful about the purposes of rules and the dicta of authority figures.

A diagnosis of antisocial personality disorder can be made only against the backdrop of behavioral information. Certain types of criminals are highly likely to produce a rash of elevations of T65 and T70 on the 10 sociopathic tendency scales. However, every respondent with this pattern of scales is not necessarily a criminal.

Special Problems

Two conditions that the psychologist is often called upon to diagnose are substance abuse and sexual difficulties. The supply of special scales fortunately contains several scales that have outstanding clinical track records in these areas.

Substance Abuse: The MacAndrew Alcoholism Scale (AMac). A number of scales have been developed from MMPI items to identify alcoholics. A 49-item scale developed by MacAndrew (1965) has rightly received the most attention.[2] Almost without exception, field tests have upheld the capacity of the AMac to distinguish male alcoholics from various nonalcoholic samples (Apfeldorf & Hunley, 1975; Rhodes, 1969; Rich & Davis, 1969; Uecker, 1970; Vega, 1971; Whistler & Cantor, 1976). Clinical experience supported by research findings indicates that AMac also identifies substance abusers in general (Burke & Marcus, 1977; Kranitz, 1972; Lachar et al., 1976, 1979) as well as substance abusers in an inactive stage either because abuse has not yet been initiated (Hoffman et al., 1974; Huber & Danahy, 1975), or because it is no longer a problem.

Views on the appropriate cutting score for AMac vary. A raw score of 24 for males is in common use, based on MacAndrew's (1965) original work supported by later independent investigations (e.g., Burke & Marcus, 1977). Lachar, Berman, Grisell, and Schooff (1976) reported that a cut-off of 23 was more efficient. Svanum, Levitt, and McAdoo (1982) recommended 25 as the cutting score based on regression analyses.

Cut-off points are always slippery matters, especially when "alcoholic–drug addict" lies on one side and "not alcoholic or drug addict" on the other. Caution must be a paramount consideration.

Means of approximately 23 have been reported for inpatient males without substance problems in several studies (e.g., Burke & Marcus, 1977; Lachar, Berman, Grisell, & Schoof, 1976). Svanum et al. (1982) reported a mean of 21.5 with an SD of 5.1. The mean AMac score for males in the Indiana normative sample is 25.08 with an SD of 4.89. Gottesman et al. (1987) reported a mean of 23 for normal 18-year-old males. Potential control guidelines thus range from around 22 to 25.

Mean scores for alcoholics have been reported as 27 (Burke & Marcus, 1977), 28 (Lachar, Berman, Grisell, & Schooff, 1976) and 30 (Svanum et al., 1982). Comparing these means with the data for possible control samples, it is plain that a cutting score of 23 or 24 will identify most of the alcoholics but with a considerable volume of false positives.

In the Burke and Marcus sample of nonsubstance abusers inpatients who were also not schizophrenic, a score of 28.2 would be T60. T60 in the Lachar et al. con-

---

2   The scale originally contained 51 items including the only 2 that deal directly with alcohol use. Conventionally, these items are not scored.

trol samples would be 28.7 for alcoholics, 28.4 for heroin addicts, and 26.2 for polydrug users. In the Svanum et al. study, 26.57 would correspond to T60 in the control sample. T60 in the Indiana sample would be a score of 29.97; it would be 27 in the Gottesman et al. sample.

There is no mathematical way to accumulate all these data so as to arrive at an absolute measure of central tendency. From inspection, it would appear that a score of 28 is a reasonable cut-off point for males. It should be pointed out, however, that cases of alcoholics with scores as low as 25 are not uncommon in clinical practice (see, for example, the case in Table 3.6).

The Svanum et al. (1982) investigation is one of the rare ones that has furnished data on female alcoholics. They reported a mean of 26.72 for alcoholics and 19.45 for a control group of inpatient nonalcoholics with a recommended cutting score of 23. The AMac mean for females in the Indiana sample is 23.32, SD = 4.58. The Gottesman et al. (1987) 18-year-old females had a mean AMac score of 20 with 24 as T60.

Evidently, there is some agreement that females in general score lower on AMac than males. A cut-off of 25 for females would appear reasonable but again, it must be noted that alcoholic females with scores of 23 and 24 are encountered in clinical practice.

Sexual Problems: The Pedophilia Scale (Pe) and the Indiana Sex Problems Scales. The Pe Scale was developed by contrasting records of 120 male pedophiles incarcerated in a California prison with 160 prisoners who had not been convicted of a sexual crime (Toobert, Bartelme, & Jones, 1959). The consequent comparison yielded 24 items that differentiated the two groups at the 5% level or beyond. These items form the Pe Scale.

Toobert et al. (1959) then proceeded to cross-validate the scale on a sample of 38 pedophiles who were not included in the original development of the scale and a group of 50 general prisoners which had also not been previously tested. A sample of 65 psychiatric patients in an Army hospital was also included in the cross-validation.

In both the original and the cross-validation study, the pedophiles scored higher on Pe than any of the other groups. The authors note that a cutting score of 8 on Pe identified approximately 75% of the pedophiles with false positives in the other groups ranging from 20 to 42%.

The Indiana normative data suggest that the cut-off is too low. The mean Pe in the Indiana sample was 6.92 with an SD of 2.46. A raw score of 10 is equivalent to T63, a status of suspicion but not certainty. T71, which would appear to be highly diagnostic, is attained by a raw score of 12.

In clinical practice, Pe has proven to be an outstandingly successful measuring instrument. Its ability to identify is not restricted to pedophiles. High scorers may also be exhibitionists or voyeurs. This is not surprising if one considers that the control groups in the developmental studies did not include paraphiliacs other than pedophiles. Thus, the Pe Scale appears to be identifying common characteristics of several groups of paraphiliacs. Examination of the scale suggests that the tendencies that are tapped by the scale are in accordance with the backward personalities of pedophiles, exhibitionists, and voyeurs as they have been unravelled in clinical examination (see for example, Gebhard, Gagnon, Pomeroy, & Christenson, 1965).

Although the Indiana Sex Problems Scale has been discussed in a previous chapter, it is presented again in its proper context. As previously noted, high scorers on I-SP are likely to have a sexual problem, often a dysfunction such as impotence, anorgasmia, sexual aversiveness, or sexual preoccupation. These different conditions are not distinguished by the scale score per se but can often be determined when I-SP is elevated from responses to individual items. For example, "Sexual things disgust me," suggests aversiveness or anorgasmia and "There is something wrong with my sexual organs," may indicate a male dysfunction.

CONFLICT

Some scales are higly positively correlated because of heavy overlap of items. An outstanding example is FAM and 4FD which have eight items in common—50% of the iems in FAM and more than 70% of 4FD. The correlation of .80 is hardly unexpected. Other scale pairs cofluctuate either positively or negatively due to the nature of the variables involved rather than to item overlap. One would expect, for example, E/Cy and 9AMO to be positively related despite no item overlap and they are (.41). On the other side of the ledger, we should find that I-De and I-Do are negatively related and they are (-.36) with only one common item, keyed differently on the two scales.

In the individual record, scale pairs that would be expected to be either positively or negatively correlated may actually be unrelated. But scale pairs are seldom related in the direction opposite to expectation in the individual record. When this occurs, we find that the respondent has a serious conflict in the area represented by the scale pair.

Values

The usual indicators of the moral–virtuous patterns are elevations of 3NA, 6N and, sometimes, the L Scale (see Chapter 5). The negatively related scale, 9AMO, would be expected to be below the normal range.

When 9AMO is also elevated, the pattern is an indication of an intense conflict in the area of moral values. The respondent is desperately seeking to maintain his/her perception of him/herself as a righteous person but at the same time, is beset by doubts that morality is warranted in an immoral society. If the respondent is a woman and I-SP is also elevated, the conflict may involve a press to act out sexually. This is especially likely to be the case if the respondent is married although the conflict is also found in single women.

Social Anxiety and Social Stimulation

Individuals who score high on 9PMA have a high optimal stimulation level, a greater than average need for involving themselves in situations that are stimulating, pleasurably exciting. A few of us drive cars very fast or climb mountains. But for most people, stimulation is social; it is provided by interrelationships, by associating with others. The high 9PMA person who has no difficulty socializing is able to satisfy his/her need for stimulation. The respondent who elevates on 9PMA but also is high on SOC and/or TSC/I and is a low scorer on 3DSA, 4SI, and/or 9IMP, has an emotionally upsetting problem. These individuals are apt to be socially maladroit and anxious, are shy, embarrass easily, are awkward in social situations, and do not make friends easily. Thus, they have difficulty in gratifying the high optimum stimulation level. This is more likely to be true when the respondent is an adult, less likely in the case of an adolescent for whom the conflict may very well become de-emphasized by further emotional development.

Hostility Control

The individual who characteristically overcontrols hostility by denial and repression is likely to elevate on OH. Typically, this person will have a low score on hostility scales, especially HOS and AUT. The individual who characteristically denies hostility perceives himself/herself as a placid individual not given to anger. In some people, the denial mechanism is faulty even though the need to overcontrol is strong. Such individuals are not only high scorers on OH but also on scales like HOS. The conflict between the need to control hostility and the need to express it is likely to be painful and is apt to be reflected in elevations on symptom scales.

Dependency–Suspicion

Dependent people rely on others to make decisions, to establish goals, and generally to assume responsibility for their lives. To be successfully dependent (bear with the contradiction in terms), one must be naive and trusting. A chronically cynical, suspicious person obviously has difficulty in establishing relationships and thus cannot fulfill dependency needs. The conflict of needs is usually experienced in late adolescence or early adulthood and brings symptoms with it.

A typical instance is the 19-year-old female college student whose T-scores on I-De and I-Do were 59 and 38 respectively—a characteristic pair of scores for the dependent person. Unfortunately, she also had scores of T59 on TSC/S, T66 on S+, and T66 on E/Cy. She came into outpatient psychotherapy with depression as presenting complaint: DEP = T75; TSC/D = T79; also I-SC = T78, and MOR = T74. At the end of a year—40 visits—her depression scores were essentially unchanged, a tribute to the suspiciousness that made it impossible for her to participate in a therapeutic alliance.

PROGNOSIS

The Control Scale (Cn)

Some seriously emotionally disturbed individuals urgently require hospitalization. Others, whose symptoms appear to be serious, maintain themselves in the community, at least marginally. How to tell the one from the other, to determine who needs (expensive) hospitalization and who does not, is a perennial clinical problem.

An MMPI approach to this problem was attempted by Cuadra (1956). Cuadra decided on a contrasting group approach, simple in conception, but tedious to carry out as carefully as Cuadra did. The first step was to select 30 young, reasonably well-educated psychiatric patients who had voluntarily sought treatment and were tested within 15 days of admission. These "criterion abnormals" were then matched with a group of "criterion normals," which was Cuadra's way of describing a group that was equally as disturbed but for whom hospitalization had not been recommended. The two groups were essentially similar in age and education and were almost identical in scores on MMPI clinical and validity scales. Cuadra had to sift through 4,000 records in order to obtain his criterion normals!

Cuadra's Control Scale (Cn) consists of 32 items which had discriminated the two criterion groups best for both sexes plus an additional 18 items which were not quite as discriminating but discriminated in the same direction for both sexes. There was little overlap in the total scale scores between Cuadra's criterion groups. The range of scores for the "normal" was 27–45; for the "abnormals" 9–33. Only four scores in the normal group were below 30; only one of the abnormals was above 30.

Forty-four of the 50 items on Cn are found on one or another of the clinical scales or the F Scale. One of the psychometric advantages of Cn is that of these 40 items, 19 are keyed in the direction opposite to the conventional scoring. Thus, an individual does not automatically elevate on Cn simply by endorsing psychopathological items.

Inspection of the scale suggests that high scorers on the scale will have a greater tendency to admit to relatively minor behavioral shortcomings and to be less religious than low scorers.

The scale can be used in accordance with its original intention, that is, low scorers with serious psychopathology should be hospitalized; high scorers (above T65) are better able to subsist on an outpatient basis. However, a high score does not necessarily rule out a "faking bad" response posture, as Cuadra originally suggested, probably because most of the items in the scale are not endorsed in the deviant direction by individuals who are faking bad.

Work Attitude Scale

A significant aspect of emotional illness, one that is sometimes neglected by diagnosticians, is the patient's subjective feeling of incapacity. Certainly there are multiple factors involved in a person's belief that he/she has lost the ability to work productively in whatever setting. Surely one of the most important is the subjective feeling that symptomatology is so overpowering that cognitive and intellectual capacities are stifled and motivation is undermined.

The Work Attitude Scale (WA; Tydlaska & Mengel, 1953) measures this feeling with reasonable accuracy. The scale was originally developed by contrasting groups of industrial employees who had received regular merit ratings of "satisfactory" over a 2-year period with a group of Air Force personnel, most of whom had gone AWOL or were disciplinary problems.

Fifty-eight items were selected by judges (not otherwise described) on the basis of estimated potential for distinguishing between the two groups. Items that dealt with sociopathic behavior such as alcohol abuse and difficulties with authorities were eliminated on the grounds that although they might very well discriminate the two groups, they would not be helpful for the purposes of the proposed scale.

MMPIs of the two groups were now examined and it was found that 37 of the 58 selected items discriminated at the 1% level. These became the Work Attitude Scale (WA). The mean WA score for the Air Force personnel was 16.4, for the industrial employees, 7.0. All but one of the former had scores above 10 while nearly 80% of the latter had scores below 10.

The scale was subsequently cross-validated on college student samples (Tesseneer & Tydlaska, 1956). Faculty members at a small state college selected 26 male students with whom they were personally familiar and whom they identified "as outstanding examples of good work attitudes." An equal number of students was selected as representing "poor work attitudes" by the faculty. The mean ages and IQs were essentially similar. The poor work attitude students were found to have a mean WA of 13.1 compared to 7.3 for the good work attitude students. The former were also found to have more psychopathology in general as measured by the clinical scales of the MMPI but, of course, this does impeach the validity of WA. It simply suggests that one effective interference with academic achievement is emotional upset.

Examination of the 37 items of WA indicates that a plurality— 10—are found on DEP and TSC/D. Somewhat smaller groups are found in 2MD and 8CON. In fact, these are exactly the components that would be anticipated for this scale: dysphoric affect, interference with cognitive processes, and lack of motivation.

Patients who score in the range T60-69 on WA are complaining that their daily life functioning is impaired to some degree but not enough to require hospitalization. Scores of T70 and above indicate that emotional disturbance is sufficiently intense so that the patient feels that he/she cannot function productively. Hospitalization or medication may be requisite, depending on the level of Cn.

Alienation and Suspicion

Patients who score high on TSC/S and/or S+, especially T70 or above, do not make "good" patients. They doubt the benevolent intentions of the psychotherapist and are unlikely to develop sufficient trust and confidence to effectuate a productive course of therapy. The prognosis is even poorer when there are accompanying elevations on the alienation scales 4SOA, 8SOA, and Ho, not unusual cofluctuations. Such individuals are cynical, demanding, and externalize blame. They resist therapeutic efforts designed to move them to assume responsibility for their own behavior. Patients with high scores on any two of these five scales have a poor prognosis with any talking therapy.

Schizoid Tendency

The patient who scores low on 3DSA, 4SI, and 9IMP and high on SOC and TSC/I will have difficulty relating to a therapist in a productive fashion. Typically, such patients have trouble communicating verbally, especially the expression of feelings. The process of therapy is slow and a therapist requires unusual patience. Patients with low scores on at least one of the social comfort scales and a high score on at least one of the social introversion scales have a guarded prognosis with talking therapies.

CHAPTER 5
THE MEASUREMENT OF
ADJUSTMENT AND PERSONALITY

It is possible that the creators of the MMPI regarded it as an all-purpose instrument that would assess personality as well as diagnose emotional disorder. The occurrence of the word "personality" itself in the title is suggestive. Perhaps the ambition was limited, a thought that might follow from the expression of purpose "to assay those traits that are commonly characteristic of disabling psychological abnormality" (Hathaway & McKinley, 1951, p.5). Mental health professionals have employed the MMPI in all ways: as a diagnostic instrument, as a measure of emotional adjustment, and as a technique for personality assessment. No matter how it is used, the major shortcoming of the MMPI clinical scales intrudes on the accuracy and utility of results. The multidimensionality of the clinical scales makes diagnosis difficult; it interferes to even a greater degree with assessment of personality and adjustment. The Harris and Lingoes scales illustrate the extent to which logical fractionation of the clinical scales improves evaluation.

High-point code typologies are of less value in personality assessment than in diagnostic evaluation, no matter what stance one assumes with respect to interpretation. Greene (1980) remarked that studies of MMPI high points have typically been restricted to scales that were T70 or above. Then what could one say about the respondent whose profile was entirely below T60?

Graham (1977) at one time adopted a radical position that overlooked the weakness of code typology. He contended that *absolute elevations* of the scales in a 2-point code are irrelevant. "A careful examination of the existing literature," claimed Graham, "suggests that in most cases the same basic extra-test behavioral correlates emerge for two-point codes irrespective of the order of the two scales and their absolute and relative elevations" (Graham, 1977, p. 64).

This concept of the 2-point pair is indefensible. Many psychologists might agree with Graham that 48/84 persons "are seen by others as odd, peculiar, and queer...their behavior is erratic and unpredictable...prostitution, promiscuity, and sexual deviation are fairly common among 48/84 individuals" (Graham, 1977, p.74; 1987, pp. 108-109). Most of those psychologists would have reference to a profile in which Scales 4 and 8 were T70 or above. One can hardly imagine a clinician who would render Graham's interpretation when the high-point pair was T60 or below. In fact, Graham has since shifted positions and currently agrees that "the descriptors presented for a particular code type are more likely to fit a subject with that code type if the two scales in the code type are elevated above T= 70" (Graham, 1987, p. 98).

High-point code typologies may have some utility when the high points are very high simply because more of the items in each scale have evoked the deviant response. Much of the elaborate library of statements that follows face validly from the content of scale items is more likely to be applicable to the respondent. The lower the scale elevations, the less probable it becomes that any set of personality and symptom descriptors will be applicable to the individual respondent.

The greater versatility and homogeneity of MMPI special scales improves personality assessment just as it does for diagnostic capacity. This chapter discusses the evaluation of some personality traits using special scales. Before that undertaking, it is obligatory to acknowledge that special scales cannot evaluate adjustment except in the restricted sense of asymptomatology. Psychologists who have some familiarity with special scales may believe otherwise. It is for this reason that the following discussion is included in this book.

THE MEASUREMENT OF PSYCHOLOGICAL ADJUSTMENT:
A FAILURE OF THE MMPI ITEM POOL

The concept of *ego strength*, or *ego resources*, or *ego control* (perhaps the best term since it indicates not only strength but implies that the ego dominates the less corticate id and superego) has been an important construct in psychological theory since the early days of Freud. The underlying notion is that the ego, the reality oriented part of the personality, successfully controls the impulses emanating from the id and the superego whose capacities to perceive reality are limited, thus a definition in effect of mental and emotional health. Few question the value of the construct in theory. So it is not surprising that one of the first special scales emerging from the MMPI pool was an Ego-Strength Scale (Es; Barron, 1953).

Barron's Es consists of 68 items that differentiated 17 outpatients at a Veterans' Administration clinic who improved with a regimen of psychotherapy from 16 patients who did not improve. Improvement ratings were made by two expert judges on the basis of available documents. From the vantage point of 25 years later, Barron's methodology appears somewhat primitive. Sophisticated researchers now view psychotherapy outcome as a dimension or a process, not a dichotomy. But there is a more compelling reason to anticipate that any effort to measure strength of ego in a meaningful way using MMPI items is doomed to failure.

There are two ways to view the ego. In one conception, the individual who is high in ego power has a superior psychological adjustment, perhaps approaching an ideal such as that of Maslow's self-actualizing person. Contemporary constructs that would be synonymous with such a level of ego are *hardiness* (Kobasa, 1979, 1982) and *high-level wellness* (Ardell, 1977; Greenberg, 1985). High-level wellness and hardiness had no place in Freudian theory. Freud believed that ego-strength enables the individual to avoid symptoms; happiness was merely the escape from pain. Hardiness has surplus meaning beyond being asymptomatic. A measure of ego-strength that was more than simply the ability to avoid symptoms could have multiple important uses. It would be an effective measure of therapy progress and outcome and a prime tool for the selection of applicants for a wide variety of professions and occupations that require maturity. Unfortunately, it is literally impossible to construct such a subinventory from the MMPI pool.

A majority of the items in the MMPI pool are symptom statements. The respondent denies the presence of symptoms by responding "false" to the item, for example:

Most of the time I wish I were dead.
I am afraid when I look down from a high place.

A smaller set of items are keyed so that a "true" response indicates denial of a symptom, for example:

I usually feel that life is worthwhile.
I do not have a great fear of snakes.

Some items allege an equivalence of health or lack of symptoms with a norm, that is, the respondent indicates that he/she is normal, for example:

I am in just as good physical health as most of my friends.
I believe I am no more nervous than most others.

A few items affirm that the respondent's current state has not suffered across time, for example:

I am about as able to work as I ever was.
My eyesight is as good as it has been for years.

Basically, these types of items, which make up the bulk of the MMPI pool, either endorse or deny symptoms, nothing more. They cannot possibly be perceived as measuring a state that is reflected in a concept like hardiness. There are no more than a half-dozen MMPI items that could, in the broadest definition, be viewed as measuring a supernormality:

I have a good appetite.
I wake up fresh and rested most mornings.
My daily life is full of things that keep me interested.
I enjoy many different kinds of play and recreation.
I am entirely self-confident.
It is great to be living in these times when so much is going on.

The appetite item is the only one of the six that is included in Es although it would hardly seem to matter since all six would constitute less than 10% of the items in Es.

Nevertheless, Es has been the most widely used special scale by clinicians (Moreland and Dahlstrom, 1983) and is one of the rare special scales that has been the subject of a fair amount of experimental scrutiny. In view of the stuff of which Es is made, it should come as no surprise that the research hardly justifies its clinical use. It is surprising that Es has received so much research attention while Block's ego-control and ego-resiliency scales (Block, 1965), also composed of MMPI items, have been largely neglected. The methodology of development of the Block scales is superior to that of Es although they are no more likely to be successful construct measures.

Studies suggesting evidence for the validity of Es are of two types: (a) emotionally disturbed persons are shown to score lower than normal people (Taft, 1957; Quay, 1955; Kleinmuntz, 1960) although not invariably (Winter & Stortroen, 1963); (b) Es distinguishes between criterion groups according to hypothesis but so do other MMPI scales or scales composed of MMPI items (e.g., King-Ellison Good, 1957; Grosz & Levitt, 1959; Van Evra & Rosenburg, 1963; Snow & Held, 1973).

Such findings are unconvincing. Any set of 68 randomly selected MMPI items would have a high probability of distinguishing between patients and normals. Significantly, Es has demonstrated poor capacity to discriminate among patients with various diagnoses associated with degrees of severity (e.g., Tamkin & Klett, 1957;

Tamkin, 1957; Sinnett, 1962; Hawkinson, 1961; Rosen, 1963; Shipman, 1965). The fact that other MMPI scales also discriminate suggests that discrimination is a function of nonspecific item content; it occurs simply because the MMPI as an instrument measures psychopathology or absence of psychopathology.

In addition to the studies already cited, evidence for lack of validity for Es is generally more convincing. Included are several unsuccessful attempts to find positive relationships between Es and Rorschach measures of ego-strength (e.g., Tamkin, 1957; Levine & Cohen, 1962; Adams & Cooper, 1962; Adams, Cooper, & Carvera 1963; Herron, Guido, & Kantor, 1965; Barger & Sechrest, 1961). Even more damaging are several investigations in which Es was unsuccessful in predicting treatment outcome (e.g., Crumpton, Cantor, & Batiste, 1960; Levine & Cohen, 1962; Hawkinson, 1961). Crumpton et al. (1960) also found that while a student sample had a higher mean Es score than a patient sample, the overlap in distributions was so great that the most predictive cut-off score—which identified 97% of the students—did no better than chance at identifying patients. These researchers add that their findings "suggest strongly that the Barron ego strength scale is misnamed. Inspection of the content reveals that the scale takes a negative approach to the measurement of ego strength, i.e., the absence of indications of ego weakness is interpreted as ego strength...'ego weakness' would be a better term of what the scale is measuring than the term 'ego strength'...the construct of ego strength should imply more than merely the absence of specific weaknesses" (Crumpton et al., 1960, p. 290).

Greene (1980) declined to provide interpretations of Es scores because "the contradictory nature of the research on the Es scale makes it inappropriate" (p.192). Archer (1987) warned that "the use of the Es scale is clearly controversial for both adults and adolescent populations, and MMPI interpreters who employ this measure should be aware that predictions from the Es scale are often likely to be misleading in term of treatment prognosis" (p.126).

In view of the nature of the MMPI item pool, the conclusions of Crumptom et al., Archer's warning, and Greene's caution were inevitable. The MMPI does not contain a subset of items that can assess psychological adjustment except in the limited sense that the term is synonymous with an absence of symptoms.

Despite the failure to measure psychological adjustment, special scales do a decent job of assessing *social* adjustment and certain personality characteristics and patterns.

THE MEASUREMENT OF SOCIAL ADJUSTMENT

There is no effective, single measure of social adjustment–maladjustment among the MMPI clinical scales although Scale 0 is often regarded as such an index. The study by deMendonca et al. (1984) shows that conventional interpretations of Scale

0 use such terms as *aloof, reserved, retiring, shy* and *withdrawn* for high scorers on this scale and *sociable, friendly* and *outgoing* for low scorers. But terms like *inhibited* and *uninhibited, self-confident, friendly, sociable,* and *withdrawn* have also been used as descriptors of high and low scorers on clinical scales other than Scale 0.

A content analysis of Scale 0 by Serkownek (Schuerger et al., 1987) suggests that it is as multifaceted as other MMPI clinical scales. Even though the dimension of social adjustment–maladjustment is very broad, some of the Serkownek subscales are not located on the dimension. This finding is consonant with some of the early studies cited in Dahlstrom, Welsh, and Dahlstrom (1972) which reported that some of the terms also used to characterize high scorers on Scale 0 were modest, sensitive, natural, serious, kind, affectionate, soft-hearted, sentimental, stereotyped, lacking originality, permissive, and generally insecure.

There are some eight special scales that have bearing on the social adjustment–maladjustment continuum. Most of these scales show item overlap and moderate to high intercorrelations.

Three Harris and Lingoes scales measure social poise and comfort; low scorers on 3DSA, 4SI, and 9IMP tend to be socially anxious and maladroit. Since there are only 26 items represented in these three scales, one must anticipate at least two elevated above T60 before a statement can be made about social anxiety. 4SI is likely to be the most reliable of the three since it has the most items.

Two other scales measure schizoid tendency: Wiggins' SOC and the Tryon, Stein, and Chu Social Introversion Scale (TSC/I). Since the item overlap amounts to more than 50% for each scale, it is expected that they will cofluctuate markedly. But as it is so often the case in the use of special scales in a pattern, it is always more convincing and thus more diagnostically warranted when more than one scale assessing in the same area is elevated.

The high scorers on SOC and TSC/I are more than socially anxious; they tend also to be self-conscious, reserved, reticent, and show a tendency to withdraw under stress. At an intermediate elevated level they are introverted; at levels of T70 and above, schizoid.

Two other scales tap the opposite end of this dimension. One is Wiggins Hypomania Scale (HYP). Those scoring in the range T60-69 are outgoing individuals who usually appear cheerful and enthusiastic. Those with scores above T70 are likely to be easily excitable, impulsive, and emotionally labile, a condition that may reflect an immaturity that could interfere with the individual's productive existence.

One last scale that has some bearing on this dimension is the Harris and Lingoes Psychomotor Acceleration subscale (9PMA). 9PMA is a measure of the degree to which the individual requires sensation and excitement in his/her life; it is highly correlated with sensation-seeking. Normal adolescents and young adults, especially males, not infrequently score above T70 on this scale. Among adults in general, scores in the range T60-69 are associated with a tendency to extroversion, a lack of discomfort in social situations, and so on. Scores below T40 suggest discomfort and a tendency to withdraw.

SOME PERSONALITY PATTERNS REFLECTED
IN SPECIAL SCALE SCORES

Conforming and Moral

American moral standards are frequently violated by Americans. The statement is so manifestly true that it hardly seems cynical. There are also substantial numbers of people—primarily living in small towns and rural areas—who weigh moral values highly and who perceive themselves as moral, virtuous, and otherwise conforming to traditional cultural standards of personal behavior. They view the world unskeptically and believe that social malignancy and evil-doers are rare.

Such respondents elevate on 3NA and 6N primarily; sometimes on 5C, REL, and/or the Lie Scale. In fact, the conforming-moral pattern is the sole explanation of the high L Scale score in a person of normal intelligence. Negatively related scale scores are invariably low, especially 9AMO and including the alienation, hostility and suspicion scales especially E/Cy, Ho, and TSC/S.

This pattern is found mostly in adult women and need include only 3NA, 6N, and 9AMO. In such cases, the respondent is mainly claiming chastity for herself. When 5C and/or L are also elevated, the sexual morality is joined by affirmation of old-fashioned American virtues like honesty, trust, sportsmanship, and conservatism. When REL is also high, there is an evident spiritual basis for the respondent's pattern.

These respondents tend to deny anger and hostility and have low scores on HOS and TSC/R, occasionally an elevation on OH. The latter is one of the indicators of sincerity as opposed to denial in the conforming-moral person. T-scores above 70 on both 3NA and 6N and L scores over 10 suggest denial; the respondent needs to present him/herself as conforming and moral but does not demonstrate it behaviorally.

Authority Conflict

Rebelliousness is indicated by high scores on 4AC and AUT. Those scoring high on AUT appear to have some awareness of their difficulty in accepting the dictates of authority figures. High scorers on 4AC have a similar difficulty with restrictions and control but seem unaware of their rebellious feelings.

The distinction in awareness of feelings between the two authority conflict scales is supported by the finding that it is not unusual for 4AC to elevate while AUT is within normal limits; the reverse is rare. The correlation between the two scales is only .30. Second, 4AC has substantial correlations with manifest hostility scales like HOS (.60), TSC/R (.49), and Ho (.76). AUT has minimal relationships with HOS (.28) and Ho (.17) and none with TSC/R.

Using adult norms, a number of normal adolescents, especially males, score in the range T65-70 on 4AC. TSC/R is sometimes also elevated. In delinquent adolescents, AUT, HOS, and Ho are also likely to be high.

Acting-Out

A high score on 9PMA ordinarily indicates a high optimum stimulation level. These individuals have a greater than normal need to have sensations, to experience excitement and will take risks to gain those experiences. They seek social, community, and sports activities and usually enjoy the company of others. The correlation of .79 with HYP is not unexpected (high 9PMA individuals low on HYP have a problem).

Scores of T60–70 are not uncommon among normal adolescents, especially males, and young adult males. Adolescents may even score above T70 without indicating serious psychopathology. However, when HOS or Ho are high, especially above T68, the prediction of hostile acting-out behavior is tenable. A potential for sexual acting-out may be inferred when Pe is above T65 in men or I-SP is elevated by either a male or female respondent.

Dependency–Dominance

Everyone has dependency and dominance needs. In most of us, the two are generally in balance and the net is unremarkable psychologically. Some individuals are overbalanced in one or the other need; such individuals are regarded as having a dependency or a dominance need that is psychologically notable. In the former instance, it is conventional to refer to a dependent personality. The consequence of a strong dominance need is not so clear since people who need to be dominant may or may not actualize that need successfully.

I-De and I-Do measure dependency need and dominance need, respectively. A respondent with I-De of T60 or above is usually classically dependent with self-esteem maintained largely extrinsically, lack of self-confidence, inability to make decisions, and a tendency to subordinate his/her needs and desires to the wishes of those on whom he/she depends. Such respondents rarely have scores on I-Do above T45 and never above T50.

TABLE 5.1
Young Adult Male Exhibitionist
Some Significant Scale Findings (T-Scores)

I-De	I-Do	TSC/I	SOC
60	15	69	72

HOS	TSC/R	Ho	TSC/S
42	45	45	39

Pe	I-SP
64	75

Individuals with I-Do scores in the range T60-69 claim to be confident, self-assured, assertive, with strong opinions and a need to dominate relationships. Scores on I-De are seldom above T45 and are usually T40 and below.

Scores above T70 on I-Do suggest that the various claims of confidence, and the like, are probably not valid. This individual seeks urgently to be dominant in interpersonal spheres but lacks the necessary positive personality characteristics to succeed.

In the mid ranges of scores on I-De and I-Do, dependency and dominance needs are usually balanced and no diagnostic statement is required. Typically, the difference between the T-scores of the two scales will not exceed +10. In some cases, the interpretation of a scale depends on the level of the other. When either I-De is above T50 and I-Do is at least T15 less, a dependency need is manifested. Similarly, if I-Do is above T50 and I-De is at least T15 less, a statement concerning dominance is warranted. These are, of course, tendencies and are not stated as definitely as when scores reach T60.

Table 5.1 presents a young male exhibitionist who can best be described as passive–dependent, suggestible, and easily manipulated. He has serious problems relating to others, is shy, embarrasses easily in social situations, and has a marked tendency to withdraw into passivity in the fact of stress. The elevations on Pe and I-SP are markers that indicate his sexual deviancy. Note that the hostility scales, HOS, Ho, and TSC/R, are all below normal and might have been expected to be even lower.

Passive–Aggressive

Dependent people need to think of themselves as agreeable and friendly; angry feelings are characteristically denied. One cannot afford hostility if one depends on others to assume one's responsibilities, make one's decisions and generally guide one's life. Thus, respondents who are judged to be dependent based on I-De and I-Do typically have low scores on hostility scales such as HOS, AUT, and Ho, like the case in Table 3.6.

We know that dependent people do harbor angry feelings and that some of them are characterized by a passive expression of that hostility in procrastination, forgetfulness, and sluggish behavior. Such individuals are often identified by scores of T60 or higher on some hostility scales, usually 4AC and/or TSC/R accompanying the I-De-I-Do imbalance that indicates the dependent person.

The Assertive Woman

The woman who scores T60 or above on Astvn is likely to be aware of her personal rights and to know something about the difference between assertiveness and aggression—but not invariably. Women with high scores on Astvn rarely have high scores on I- De—the correlation is -.51, an understandable finding. Neither do they tend to have scores above T60 on I-Do; the correlation is minimal .30. Rather, they fall into the group that ranges from T40 to T59 with I-Do higher than I-De.

A critical score is FEM which is unrelated to Astvn. Respondents with scores in the normal range of FEM are the appropriately assertive women. Those with low scores on FEM, especially lower than T40, are more likely to be aggressive rather than assertive and to give indications of rejecting a feminine gender identity. Not infrequently, I-SP will be elevated; examination of the items in this scale may reveal deviant responses to item 74 ("I have never been sorry that I am a girl"), and/or item 470 ("Sexual things disgust me").

The hostility scales are also relevant. TSC/R has a small, negative correlation (-.26) with Astvn. The other hostility scales are unrelated. The assertive woman who does not have a problem with gender identity will usually have hostility scales within the normal range. Elevations on the hostility scales are another indicator of the woman who is having a gender identity problem.

CHAPTER 6
MMPI SPECIAL SCALES
AND THE RORSCHACH

Surveys over the years have shown that the MMPI and the Rorschach are two of the most frequently used diagnostic instruments in mental health facilities (Sundberg, 1961; Lubin, Larsen, & Matarazzo, 1983; Wade & Baker, 1977).[1] The common assumption is that each measures psychopathology and taps personality trends but from a different direction, as might be expected of an objective and a projective test. A further assumption is that the MMPI draws on the respondent's conscious view of himself/herself while the Rorschach taps tendencies that exist below the level of the subject's conscious awareness. Thus, the common joint usage of these two instruments is understandable.

OVERVIEW OF THE EARLY CORRELATIONAL STUDIES

In view of their popularity, one might expect that there would be considerable interest in the formal relationship between the MMPI and the Rorschach. Certainly appropriate correlational studies have the potential for many interesting findings that might have broad bearing on personality theory and psychopathology.

---

1   It is assumed that the reader is familiar with Rorschach scoring and interpretation. If in doubt, the reader is advised to consult any basic Rorschach reference book, such as Levitt (1980a).

It is somewhat disappointing to discover that there have been only a handful of such investigations over the past 40 years, an average of less than one per year. Perhaps this is a consequence of the fact that most psychologists who are interested in the MMPI are disinterested in the Rorschach and vice versa although their joint popularity makes this somewhat difficult to believe.

As a group, the Rorschach–MMPI correlational investigations are methodologically flawed and have generally yielded conflicting or negative results, for example, Dana and Bolton (1982); Smith and Coyle (1969); Forsyth (1959); Rice (1968); Zimet and Brackbill (1956); Rosen (1952); Blanton and Landsman (1952); Clark (1948); Williams and Lawrence (1954); Leavitt and Garron (1982); and Cutter (1957). Several of these investigations utilized a group Rorschach technique which limits the information that is yielded by this instrument (Rice, 1968; Branton & Landsman, 1952; Thompson, 1948; Clark, 1948). Most of the investigations tested specific hypotheses and several did have positive results. For some reason, there seem to be an interest in relating Barron's Ego-Strength Scale (Es) (Barron, 1953) to allegedly comparable Rorschach indices such as those that depend on accuracy of responses. Most of these studies had negative results.

Among positive findings, Goodstein and Goldberger (1955) found that 5 of 17 Rorschach indices differentiated groups of college students defined as high and low on anxiety on the basis of the Manifest Anxiety Scale (Taylor, 1953), which is composed of MMPI items. The variables included anxiety and hostility content and the use of dark color. However, 4 of these factors were significant on the basis of one-tailed tests whose application is questionable.

Tamkin (1957) reported significant negative correlations between F+% and the F Scale and a set of critical items devised by Grayson (1951). Taulbee (1961) found a significant correlation between flexor movement responses and Scales 2 and 7 of the MMPI. He found no relationship with the overall number of movement responses which fitted with his hypothesis that flexor M responses reflect lack of mental health. Adams et al. (1963) found that only Scale 5 had a significant correlation with the Rorschach Prognostic Rating Scale (Klopfer, Kirkner, Wisham, & Baker, 1954).

Thompson (1948) reported that among her college students subjects, a subgroup that had Dd responses with movement showed greater elevations on seven MMPI clinical scales compared to students who did not have such Rorschach responses although none of the differences were statistically significant.

Rice, Slembach, and Pann (1969) attempted to use the entire protocol through the employment of expert judges. Instead of correlating factors with scales, three judges were asked to place the subject in a diagnostic category on the basis of both the Rorschach and the MMPI separately: neurotic, organic, personality disorder, or psychotic. The agreement between the two instruments for the three judges was 70%, 75%, and 84% of the pairs of tests for 100 randomly selected patients. Over the three judges, the frequency of agreement on diagnostic impression was significantly greater for the MMPI than for the Rorschach.

In some of the aforementioned studies, the protocols were taken from clinical hospital records. In others, it is unclear whether the Rorschach records were obtained by a single examiner or by multiple examiners. In some instances, the scoring system is not clear. Almost none of the reports make any reference to an attempt to standardize the administration of the Rorschach. Except for Es and occasionally another special scale, the investigations limited themselves to the standard MMPI clinical and validity scales.

The Reading and Haymond Studies

There have been two, relatively recent, unpublished works which manifest greater methodological rigor and which examined many MMPI special scales (Reading, 1978; Haymond, 1981). In each of these investigations, a standard method of administering the Rorschach was employed with each subject (Levitt, 1980a), all of the records were obtained and scored by the same examiner and the MMPIs were scored for a large number of special scales. The administrative standardization attempted to eliminate the examiner factor from the Rorschach data while the special scales made possible a relatively wide varity of hypotheses.

Each study suffered from some unfortunate weaknesses, nevertheless. The Reading study used only 25 subjects after discarding an unknown number because the Rorschach inquiries were inadequate for scoring. In some cases, the MMPI was given first, in others, the Rorschach.

The Haymond study had an N of 100 and none were discarded for any reason. In every case, the MMPI was administered approximately 10 days prior to the Rorschach. Haymond's sample, while respectable in size, is narrow in scope since it was composed entirely of females between the ages of 12 and 18 who had been referred to a juvenile diagnostic center. The sample had a mean IQ of 92 and the reading comprehension in the group required that the MMPI be administered to some subjects by means of a cassette tape.

Despite the defects of these investigations they are worth examining.

Es did poorly in both investigations. Haymond found no relationship between Es and Rorschach measures of adjustment like F+%, XF+%, M, or FC. Reading reported a *positive correlation* between F- and Es and a *negative relationship* between F+ and Es.

Earlier investigations had hinted at the possibility that Rorschach content rather than formally scored factors might be more related to MMPI scales. This turned out to be the case to some extent in the Reading thesis. Two such Rorschach factors had understandable correlations with a large number of MMPI special scales. They were *perseveration* and *sex content*. Perseveration is the senseless repetition of a response through the Rorschach card deck.

The match between the shape of the object and the shape of the blot is fairly
accurate when the response is first given; when the response is repeated in
subsequent cards, however, the form of the blot is forced into the form of the
object, in almost complete disregard of the actual form properties of the blots,
the object, or both. (Klopfer & Spiegelman, 1956, p. 285)

While perseveration is regarded as a sign of serious psychopathology—
schizophrenia or organic brain damage—sex content is usually thought of as a
reflection of anxiety and a neurotic adjustment (Goldfried, Stricker, & Weiner
1971). Beck, for example, considered Sx (the number of responses with sex as
content) as an indicator of free-floating anxiety although he also suggested that it
might reflect a serious regression (Beck, 1952).

In the Reading study, Sx had significant positive correlations ranging from .41
to .65 with 10 indices of psychopathology including I-RD, I-DS, PSY, and PHO;
positive correlations ranging from .46 to .58 with seven measures of sociopathy
such as Ho, HOS and 4SOA. In addition, the obvious hypothesis of a relationship
between Sx and I-SP was validated by a coefficient of .56.

The occurence of perseveration had positive correlations ranging from .40 to
.78 with six measures of psychopathology including I-RD and PSY and positive
coefficients ranging from .43 to .57 with seven measures of sociopathy including
Ho, 9AMO and AMac. The obvious hypothesis of a relationship with I-OC was
supported by a correlation coefficient of .55. It should be noted that the anatomy
response, generally considered to be an indicator of psychopathology on the
Rorschach, was unrelated to MMPI indices of psychopathology including most of
the health concerns scales.

In the Haymond study, most of the significant correlation coefficients were
between .20 and .30, fairly small compared to those in the Reading thesis.
However, they are not unexpected in view of the homogeneity of Haymond's
population. Among Haymond's data, Sx and perseveration do not stand out. They
were totally unrelated to MMPI indices of psychopathology, mostly due to the fact
that their means were very close to zero. Another Rorschach index of
psychopathology—*contaminatory tendency*—was significantly positively related
to seven MMPI psychopathology scales including I-RD and PSY. A contamination is the fusion of two incompatible objects into a single, peculiar, or bizarre percept. By unanimous clinical consensus, it is a hallmark of the schizophrenic
respondent. A contaminatory tendency—what Exner (1986) called an Inappropriate Combination—is a sort of minor contamination in that the alien objects
are in different parts of the blot, such as "a person with the head of a chicken." Contaminatory tendency occurs in the Rorschach records of normal respondents but it
occurs almost twice as often in the records of psychiatric outpatients and nearly
four times as frequently in the records of psychiatric inpatients (Exner, 1978).

Haymond had some other interesting findings. For example, figure-ground reversal, usually considered to be a Rorschach indicator of negativism and hostility, was significantly related to HOS, AUT, and 9AMO. XF+%, generally considered to be the best indicator of adjustment on the Rorschach, had expected negative correlations with I-RD, I-DS, and 8BSE. The alienation scales 4SOA and 8SOA had significant negative relationships with H%, the percent of human responses in the Rorschach record, again not unexpectedly. Cn had a significant positive relationship with M, the number of movement responses, as might be expected from the clinical interpretation of Cn. Similarly, 5C had a significant relationship with P, the number of popular responses on the Rorschach, usually considered to be a mark of attunement to the demands of conventionality. As in the Reading thesis, the anatomy response was unrelated to MMPI measures of psychopathology including health concern scales.

Many of the hypotheses that were tested in the Reading and Haymond works were not supported by their data. However, there is enough in the way of positive findings, despite the methodological shortcomings of these studies, to suggest strongly that the Rorschach is supporting the validity of its old team mate— to use the metaphor employed in the title of Haymond's dissertation— at least insofar as special scales are concerned.

CONJOINT USE OF THE RORSCHACH AND THE MMPI

The MMPI and the Rorschach are commonly employed together in various clinical settings. The two instruments frequently complement each other to improve effectiveness and accuracy of assessment. The MMPI furnishes a greater variety of data on symptoms and personality traits. The Rorschach has the advantage of unfakability and thus has the capacity to distinguish between MMPI records that are the result of response sets and other misleading circumstances.

There is no shortage of cases, especially in forensic psychology, of faking bad MMPI records with an ME of T75 and greater that have companion Rorschach profiles that are clearly within normal limits. XF+% is between 75 and 90, P is at least 5 and pathological content and other qualitative indicators of a thought disorder are absent. Or, DEP and/or TSC/D are substantially elevated but the respondent pays no attention to the dark coloration in the blots. This anomaly is not unusual in a patient who is loudly proclaiming unhappiness and dissatisfaction with the current life space and is demanding help but is not clinically depressed.

On the other side of the coin, there are some seriously disturbed individuals who are able to exercise sufficient control when presented with a structured stimulus so that they produce minimally abnormal, or even normal, MMPI records. The amorphous ink blots, however, are likely to evoke unmistakable psychopathology. For example, $XF+\%$ and P may be low while the percentage of anatomy and

TABLE 6.1
Conjoint Use of the MMPI and Rorschach

MMPI Data					Rorschach Data			
ME	PSY	I-RD	TSC/T	DEP	XF+%	P	An%	Qualitative Signs
59	52	46	51	48	50	2	36	present

From records of a 37-year-old, white, male, inpatient, obtained 4 days apart. The qualitative signs of thought disorder on the Rorschach included vagueness, loose associations and confabulation.

sex responses may be high and qualitative indicators of thought disorder such as contamination, confabulation, loose associations, and bizarre content, may be present. Table 6.1 presents some contrasting MMPI and Rorschach data from the records of a 37-year-old white male inpatient whose only complaints were physical as evidenced by substantial elevations on TSC/B, ORG, and 8BSE. The patient was something of a medical mystery; his physical complaints had persisted over a number of years and were complicated by side effects of prescribed drugs.

Table 6.1 illustrates the absence of psychopathology in the MMPI record and the testimony to an underlying psychotic process by Rorschach data.

While the Rorschach is used not infrequently to correct a specious impression created by the MMPI, the two are also often used conjointly, either providing support for each other or complementary information. Three relevant case presentations follow.

The Case of DM

DM was a 27-year-old, white, married female with a high school education who had recently assumed a managerial position with a supermarket chain. She was referred to a Chronic Pelvic Pain Clinic operated by the Department of Obstetrics & Gynecology of a large metropolitan hospital. Typically, referrals were from physicians in the community in cases where multiple diagnostic procedures did not uncover an appropriate etiology for the patient's clinical symptoms.

Examination at the CPP Clinic disclosed a previously undiscovered organic basis for the presenting complaint in an occasional patient. The vast majority of the CPP clinic patients, however, turned out to have a psychogenic basis for their symptoms as evidenced by multiple minor physical complaints and emotional symptoms, especially problems of sexual identity or sexual function. Case DM was one of the few who did not fit the psychogenic pattern and medical staff were advised to look further for organic causes. Eventually, a previously undetected tumor was found and removed.

Three years later, the lady was referred to the Psychiatry Department at another metropolitan hospital by the Rheumatology Department, needing to find some reason for persistent and progressive pains described as polyarthralgias and chronic right-sided weakness. On the occasion of this admission, a Rorschach was added to the MMPI.

What follows is a point-by-point description of the conjoint interpretation of the Rorschach and the MMPI. Note especially that both instruments are required not only to support certain diagnostic aspects but to demonstrate the unusual degree of self-deception practiced by the patient.

1. The MMPI record is valid in the sense that the respondent understood the items and responded consistently (TR and Cl both zero).

2. Patient is not seriously emotionally disturbed (XF+% = 84; P = 5; no qualitative indicators of an underlying thought process; PSY = T39; no scorable response on I-RD).

3. But she is nevertheless a chronically unhappy woman who is engaged in a massive denial of a number of unacceptable conditions. Hostility: OH = T68 and HOS = T38, Ho = T38, TSC/R = T35, that is, the respondent denies and represses hostile feelings. This interpretation is supported by 10% anatomy responses in the Rorschach content (i.e., bony anatomy = repressed hostility; Depression: DEP and TSC/D had raw scores of zero). Such remarkably low scores alone suggest denial.In addition, YF, a depression indicator, appeared among the Rorschach determinants, and D-S = T61—at least a chronic,low-grade depression is indicated; Dependency: I-Do = T51 and I-De = T29, a pair of scores that ordinarily suggests a self-assured person with low dependency needs. But three FY on the Rorschach is a clear dependency indicator, especially with two of them scored minus for response-quality—a sign of conflict in the area; Anxiety: TSC/T=T27 and PHO had no scorable responses, again the unusually low scores pointing to denial. Also, the presence of FY- in the Rorschach record suggests that anxiety accompanies conflict; Gender Identity: FEM = T42 and Astvn = T60, the combination appears to represent a woman who is not typically feminine. However, the Rorschach content was heavily feminine including such responses as women cooking or dancing, flowers, and fountains.

4. The patient perceives herself as moral, virtuous, and ingenuous (3NA = T69; 6N = T62; also E/Cy = 37 and 9AMO = 45). She claims to endorse basic American cultural values (5C = T75; L = T63).

5. She is comfortable with people, makes friends easily and enjoys social interaction (3DSA = T65; 4SI = T62 and 9IMP = T65; Rorschach Human % = 15; no depersonalized human responses; H greater than Hd).

The full report read as follows:

> The patient is defensive in her general approach to mental investigation and makes extensive use of denial. She is not psychotic though it is likely that she is denying depression and anxiety.

The testing reveals several important conflicts. The patient has a very feminine aspect to her personality which is characterized by passive-dependency and a naive view of the world in which she perceives herself as moral, virtuous and stereotypically feminine. These characteristics are apparently making it difficult for the patient to maintain her managerial role in which males are both peers and subordinates. Thus, she denies her dependency needs and attempts to be hard, assertive and masculine. The intra-psychic struggle is further complicated by the fact that the patient has difficulty expressing hostility which she characteristically denies and represses.

The patient is socially comfortable and gregarious which, along with her inability to express hostility, serve her dependency needs well. However, since her comfort in relating socially is as a female, this aspect of the personality does not lend to her performance as a manager.

The patient's conflict has become so intense that she finds a temporary resolution by developing psychogenic physical complaints. Three years ago, an organic condition served the same purpose for her. Indeed, that experience may well have been the basis on which the current symptomatology was developed. In each case, the patient was incapacitated and unable to work for considerable periods of time, extricating herself temporarily from her identity-occupational conflict.

It appears that the patient is more comfortable as the stereotyped woman. Outpatient psychotherapy is recommended in which the therapist should explore the patient's occupational goals thoroughly.

The Case of SV

SV was a 38-year-old, white, married female, a college graduate, who was seen as an outpatient. On clinical examination, the patient appeared somewhat depressed but not nearly to a degree to account for the frequency of crying episodes. The patient's mood was dysphoric but she appeared to be functioning adequately.

The conjoint analysis follows:

1. The record is considered to be valid in that the patient's comprehension was adequate (TR = 0; Cl = 3, the latter most likely the result of indecision rather than inadequate comprehension or confusion in a college education person). However, the ME of 76 with four K-corrected clinical scales above T80 strongly indicates that this is a typical "cry for help" record in which the symptom picture is exaggerated.

2. The patient is very unhappy with her life space at the moment but she is not clinically depressed although DEP = T86 and TSC/D = T94. There are three morbid responses in the Rorschach content (all squashed animals) which contribute to the impression of some dysphoria. However, notably D-S = T50 and the Rorschach record contains six color responses including four that are FC+ and no achromatic color determination, all going counter to the presence of depression.

3. As usual, the exaggeration of symptoms is accomplished with anxiety and depression scales. The patient wants it to be known that she is very disturbed but not psychotic. Thus, I-RD = T45, I-DS = T48 and PSY = T55. The Rorschach picture actually seems a bit more disturbed with XF+% = 59 and P = 4, low for a response total of 27. Blood is found in two of the squashed animal responses and there is a third blood response that is Pure C. All told, there is enough to suggest that the patient is indeed beset by anxiety and depression though her exaggeration makes it difficult to determine the extent of either symptom.

4. The patient's personality has a marked obsessive-compulsive quality as evidenced by I-OC = T60 and Rorschach Dd% = 11. The latter is not as revealing as some of the patient's remarks during the administration, such as "I don't want to bias the inkblots by sex," "I'm concerned about doing this, to get the most out of it," "the drawing appears awkward," "I hate for this to be put down on paper," but "I want to be honest," "I panic when I can't think."

5. The patient has strong dependency needs (I-De = T70 and I-Do = 38; supporting Rorschach content includes a lamb, a smile, "little bugs," and "two hands reaching out").

6. The patient describes her family atmosphere as highly unpleasant (4FD = T80 and FAM = T66 despite the fact that the patient omitted five items that appear on one or the other of these scales).

7. The patient has a serious problem with gender identity and very likely with sexual behavior itself. The indicators of these three phenomena are salient in both test instruments. To begin with, FEM = T39 which is not all that indicative in a college-educated woman especially along with Astvn = T43. But I-SP = T97. The patient endorsed the item "Sexual things disgust me" and did not respond to the item "I am strongly attracted by members of my own sex." The patient gave six sex responses, an enormous number in a Rorschach record of any length. Furthermore, two of them were penises, a more psychopathological response because of its relative infrequency compared to female genitalia responses. The patient's Pure C response was "someone having a period." She remarked in the inquiry "I am not pleased at being a female." The patient perceived the popular female figures on Card VII. On Card VIII she began by saying "Every place where there's a fold— I can see this must be a drawing of female sexual—"and in the inquiry, she noted that she had seen female genitalia on Card VII as well but had suppressed the response. She remarked spontaneously that "It sounds gay to see two women and then a vulva."

8. The patient's family difficulties and her problems with gender identity have led her to feel isolated, different, misunderstood, and lacking a social support system (4SOA = T70; 8SOA = T84; Ho = T70). Hostility is typically expressed in resentment and irritability (TSC/R = T66); the patient has difficulty expressing aggression in a more mature fashion (HOS = T58).

The text of the complete report follows:

Most of the symptom picture is obtained from the MMPI which shows clear evidence of exaggeration. The symptom picture should, therefore, be viewed with extreme caution and is presented here only for purposes of completion of the report. The patient reports herself to be high anxiety-prone and chronically tense with multiple phobias. She feels extremely unhappy and guilt ridden but is not clinically depressed. A major problem appears to be cognitive retardation; the patient reports that her memory is poor and that she cannot concentrate or think logically and clearly. This deficit apparently occurs whenever the patient feels stressed. Crying appears to be a learned stress reaction and does not necessarily indicate dysphoric mood. Even the patient's occasional suicidal urge is more likely to have been motivated by obsessive–compulsive tendencies rather than by extreme depression. The patient also reports minor physical complaints of the type usually associated with emotional illness such as vague pains, easy fatiguability, and general malaise. The patient has strong feelings of isolation, of being different and misunderstood and socially unsupported. These feelings are probably a consequence of frustration of strong dependency needs. The consequent hostility is expressed in an adolescent fashion by negativism and irritability since the patient has difficulty expressing hostility in a more adult fashion.

The patient is acutely unhappy with her family situation. She views the family milieu as quarrelsome, unpleasant, lacking in affection, overcontrolling, and infantilizing. It is most probable that these perceptions are attributable to her husband whom she blames for the frustration of her dependency needs. The patient's husband may have become alienated himself because the patient has a serious problem in gender identity which likely expresses itself in sexual behavior as well. She appears to reject heterosexual love and the stereotyped female role. She lacks many ordinary feminine interests and consciously wished that she were not a woman. Nevertheless, she appears preoccupied by sex. There is a good possibility of an underlying homosexual tendency of which the patient herself appears to have some awareness.

The Case of CI

The patient was an 18-year-old, single, white, outpatient male. He had contracted a minor illness which kept him from school for a week. After remission of symptoms, he had simply declined to leave his home and had not done so for a year and a half. He read and watched television and seemed totally unmotivated to do anything else despite various attempts at remediation by his parents. The referring psychiatrist requested information about the possibility of a schizoid personality or underlying thought disorder and the nature and extent of the patient's fantasy level.

The conjoint analysis follows:

1. The record was considered to be valid in that the patient comprehended the test items and responded truthfully to the best of his ability (TR = 1; Cl = 1; ME = 59).

2. The patient is clearly not psychotic nor is there any evidence of an underlying thought disorder (I-RD = T46; PSY = T48; XF+% = 83; P = 5; no sex, anatomy, morbid, or blood responses and no qualitative indicators of thought disorder).

3. There is no evidence of either anxiety or depression (TSC/T = T40; PHO = T40; TSC/D = T45; DEP = T40; no YF and no content indicators).

4. There is some guilt present (the lone FC is minus).

5. The patient is heavily given to fantasy, not all of which is mature but none seems to be regressive or paranoid (six M+ and three AM responses, almost 70% of the response total; there are no paranoid indicators or ideation in the Rorschach and TSC/S = T37 with I-RD = T46).

6. The patient is a passive–dependent personality characterized by an acute lack of energy or need for stimulation (I-De = T75 and I-Do = T45; FY = 3 and there is a repeated use of the word "little" in the Rorschach record; 9PMA = T37, remarkably low for an 18-year-old male; HYP = T38 which lends support to the interpretation of passivity and adds a quality of stolidity to the personality picture).

7. The patient denies that he is socially uncomfortable (3DSA = T62; 4SI = T59; 9IMP = T49) and also denies that he tends to withdraw under stress (TSC/I = T41 and SOC = T43); the Rorschach supports the patient's perception of himself (H% = 31).

8. The patient has limited ability to express hostility and some tendency to deny and repress it (HOS = T45; AUT = T37; TSC/R = T41, all very low for an 18-year-old male; and OH = T55, suggestive although not definitive).

9. The patient has stereotypic feminine interests in the extreme (FEM = T65; feminine Rorschach content—music, botany, and dancing responses).

10. Not surprisingly, the patient acknowledges that he has a sex problem although he denies that it is homosexuality and it does not appear to be a paraphilia (I-SP = T74 but Pe = T46 and there are no diagnostic critical items; no sex content on the Rorschach suggests that the patient's sexual problem is conscious and not overwhelming).

11. The patient describes himself as moral and virtuous, specifically endorsing traditional national ideals with the exception of religion which is strongly and specifically rejected (6N = T61; 3NA = T64, both unusually high for an 18-year-old male; 5C = T70 but REL = T33).

12. Family problems are denied but there is some indication of difficulty with his mother (4FD = T48; FAM = T52 but the only female percept on the Rorschach is a witch, "devious, doing something, I can't tell what").

The text of the complete report follows:

The patient is not psychotic and there is no evidence of an underlying thought disorder or of paranoid or regressive ideation. The patient does not seem to have a problem either with anxiety or depression though he has some guilt feelings, probably related to hostility toward his mother.

The basic personality structure is passive-dependent and would probably be more appropriate for a female than a male. The life style and interests are typically feminine. The patient lacks conventional masculine ambitions and is somewhat naive and trusting in his interpersonal relationships. Despite his lack of ambition, he places a high value on traditional American ideals except for religion which is strongly rejected for some idiosyncratic reason.

The patient tends to deny hostility and his optimum stimulation level is low for an adolescent male; he is somewhat retarded psychomotorically.

The patient acknowledges that he has a sex problem but its specific nature is unclear. He denies that he is a homosexual despite the strong feminine interest pattern. There is no evidence that the patient has a paraphilia of any kind. This is an area which requires further exploration.

The patient, despite his withdrawal from the community, is probably socially comfortable though it is equally probable that he lacks sufficient motivation or drive to build a social support system. Certainly he could not be characterized as a schizoid personality.

The patient appears to have some resentment toward his mother though it is denied. The resentment may have sprung up recently, a reaction to the fact that his mother accepted his unconventional behavior for a long time but now sees him as in need of professional intervention.

A plausible hypothesis is that the patient's withdrawal from the community is a function of his recognition of his personality inversion. The purpose of the withdrawal is to escape rejection and ridicule.

Appendix I

Special Scales: Descriptors, Acronyms, and Item Composition

ITEM COMPOSITION OF THE SPECIAL SCALES

Wiggins Content Scales*

SOC — Social Maladjustment
True: 52, 171, 172, 180, 201, 267, 292, 304, 377, 384, 453, 455, 509
False: 57, 91, 99, 309, 371, 391, 449, 450, 479, 482, 502, 520, 521, 547

DEP — Depression
True: 41, 61, 67, 76, 94, 104, 106, 158, 202, 209, 210, 217, 259, 305, 337, 338, 339, 374, 390, 396, 413, 414, 487, 517, 518, 526, 543
False: 8, 79, 88, 207, 379, 407

FEM — Feminine Interests
True: 70, 74, 77, 78, 87, 92, 126, 132, 140, 149, 203, 261, 295, 463, 538, 554, 557, 562
False: 1, 81, 219, 221, 223, 283, 300, 423, 434, 537, 552, 563

MOR — Poor Morale

True: 84, 86, 138, 142, 244, 321, 357, 361, 375, 382, 389, 395, 397, 398, 411, 416, 418, 431, 531, 549, 555
False: 122, 264

REL — Religious Fundamentalism
True: 58, 95, 98, 115, 206, 249, 258, 373, 483, 488, 490
False: 491

AUT — Authority Conflict
True: 59, 71, 93, 116, 117, 118, 124, 250, 265, 277, 280, 298, 313, 316, 319, 406, 436, 437, 446
False: 294

PSY — Psychoticism
True: 16, 22, 24, 27, 33, 35, 40, 48, 50, 66, 73, 110, 121, 123, 127, 136, 151, 168, 184, 194, 197, 200, 232, 275, 278, 284, 291, 293, 299, 312, 317, 334, 341, 345, 348, 349, 350, 364, 400, 420, 433, 448, 476, 511, 551
False: 198, 347, 464

ORG — Organic Symptoms
True: 23, 44, 108, 114, 156, 159, 161, 186, 189, 251, 273, 332, 335, 541, 560

---

*Source: Wiggins, 1966. (Copyright 1966 by the American Psychological Association. Reprinted by permission).

95

False: 46, 68, 103, 119, 154, 174,
175, 178, 185, 187, 188, 190,
192, 243, 274, 281, 330, 405,
496, 508, 540

FAM — Family Problems
True: 21, 212, 216, 224, 226, 239,
245, 325, 327, 421, 516
False: 65, 96, 137, 220, 527

HOS — Manifest Hostility
True: 28, 39, 80, 89, 109, 129, 139,
145, 162, 218, 269, 282, 336,
355, 363, 368, 393, 410, 417,
426, 438, 447, 452, 468, 469,
495, 536
False: None

PHO — Phobias
True: 166, 182, 351, 352, 360, 365,
385, 388, 392 473, 480, 492,
494, 499, 525, 553
False: 128, 131, 169, 176, 287, 353,
367, 401, 412, 522, 539

HYP — Hypomania
True: 13, 134, 146, 181, 196, 228,
234, 238, 248, 266, 268, 272,
296, 340, 342, 372, 381, 386,
409, 439, 445, 465, 500, 505,
506
False: None

HEA — Poor Health
True: 10, 14, 29, 34, 72, 125, 279,
424, 519, 544
False: 2, 18, 36, 51, 55, 63, 130,
153, 155, 163, 193, 214, 230,
462, 474, 486, 533, 542

Composition of Tryon, Stein, and Chu Cluster Scales*

I — Social Introversion
True: 52, 86, 138, 171, 172, 180,
201, 267, 292, 304, 317, 321,
371, 377, 509
False: 57, 79, 264, 309, 353, 415,
449, 479, 482, 521, 541

*Source: Stein, 1968. (Reprinted with permission of the author.)

II — Body Symptoms
True: 10, 14, 23, 29, 44, 47, 62, 72,
108, 114, 125, 161, 189, 191,
263, 544
False: 2, 3, 18, 36, 51, 55, 68, 103,
153, 160, 163, 175, 190, 192,
230, 243, 330

III — Suspicion
True: 71, 89, 112, 136, 244, 265,
278, 280, 284, 316, 319, 348,
368, 383, 390, 404, 406, 426,
436, 438, 447, 455, 469, 509,
558
False: None

IV — Depression
True: 41,; 61, 67, 76, 84, 104, 142,
168, 236, 259, 301, 339, 357,
361, 384, 396, 397, 411, 414,
418, 487, 526, 594
False: 8, 46, 88,107, 379

V — Resentment
True: 28, 39, 94,97, 106, 129, 139,
145, 147, 148, 162, 234, 336,
375, 381, 382, 416, 443, 468,
536
False: 399

VI — Autism
True: 15, 31, 33, 40, 100, 134, 241,
297, 329, 342, 345, 349, 356,
358, 359, 374, 389, 425, 459,
511, 545, 559, 560
False: None

VII — Tension
True: 13, 22, 32, 43, 102, 158, 166,
182, 186, 217, 238, 303, 322,
335, 337, 338, 340, 351, 360,
365, 388, 431, 439, 442, 448,
473, 492, 4949, 499, 506, 543,
555
False: 131, 152, 242, 407

Composition of Indiana Rational Scales

I-De — Dependency Inventory
True: 141, 143, 165, 398, 531, 564
False: 170, 235, 501

I-Ds — Disassociation Inventory
  True: 22, 50, 156, 194, 251, 345,
    420
  False: 464
I-Do — Dominance Inventory
  True: 79, 112, 170, 235, 257, 264,
    404, 415, 426, 432, 447, 502,
    520
  False: 82, 444, 503, 509
I-OC — Obsessive-Compulsive
  True: 64, 213, 343, 346, 358, 359,
    414, 461, 462
  False: None
I-SC — Self-Concept Inventory
  True: 74, 84, 86, 142, 209, 418, 517
  False: 73, 74, 122, 257, 262, 264
I-RD — Severe Distortion of Reality
Inventory
  True: 27, 33, 48, 50, 66, 121, 123,
    151, 184, 200, 275, 291, 334,
    345, 349, 350, 476
  False: 464
I-SP — Sex Problems Inventory
  True: 69, 85, 179, 297, 320, 470,
    519, 548*, 558*
  False: 20, 37, 74, 133, 430

Composition of Harris & Lingoes Subscales*†

Scale 2 — Depression

D_1 — Subjective Depression
  True: 32, 42, 43, 52, 67, 86, 104,
    138, 142, 158, 159, 182, 189,
    236, 259
  False: 2, 8, 46, 57, 88, 107, 122,
    131, 152, 160, 191, 207, 208,
    242, 272, 285, 296
D_2 — Psychomotor Retardation
  True: 41, 52, 182, 259
  False: 8, 30, 39, 57, 64, 89, 95, 145,
    207, 208, 233

D_3 — Physical Malfunctioning
  True: 130, 189, 193, 288
  False: 2, 18, 51, 153, 154, 155, 160
D_4 — Mental Dullness
  True: 32, 41, 86, 104, 159, 182, 259,
    290
  False: 8, 9, 46, 88, 122, 178, 207
D_5 — Brooding
  True: 41, 67, 104, 138, 142, 158,
    182, 236
  False: 8, 107

Scale 3 — Hysteria

Hy_1 — Denial of Social Anxiety
  True: None
  False: 141, 172, 180, 201, 267, 292
Hy_2 — Need for Affection
  True: 253
  False: 26, 71, 89, 93, 109, 124, 136,
    162, 234, 265, 289
Hy_3 — Lassitude-Malaise
  True: 32, 43, 76, 189, 238
  False: 2, 3, 8, 9, 51, 107, 137, 153,
    160, 163
Hy_4 — Somatic Complaints
  True: 10, 23, 44, 47, 114, 186
  False: 7, 55, 103, 174, 175, 188, 190,
    192, 230, 243, 274
Hy_5 — Inhibition of Aggression
  True: None
  False: 6, 12, 30, 128, 192, 147, 170

Scale 4 — Psychopathic Deviate

Pd_1 — Familial Discord
  True: 21, 42, 212, 216, 224, 245
  False: 96, 137, 235, 237, 527
Pd_2 — Authority Problems
  True: 38, 59, 118, 520
  False: 37, 82, 141, 173, 289, 294,
    429
Pd_3 — Social Imperturbability
  True: 64, 479, 520, 521
  False: 82, 141, 171, 180, 201, 267,
    304, 352
Pd_{4A} — Social Alienation
  True: 16, 24, 35, 64, 67, 94, 110,
    127, 146, 239, 244, 284, 305,

---

*Source: Harris & Lingoes (1955/rev. 1968).

†Scored for male respondents only

368, 520
False: 20, 141, 170
Pd$_{4B}$—Self-Alienation
  True: 32, 33, 61, 67, 76, 84, 94,
    102, 106, 127, 146, 215, 368
  False: 8, 107

Scale 6—Paranoia

Pa$_1$—Persecutory Ideas
  True: 16, 24, 35, 10, 121, 123, 127,
    151, 157, 202, 275, 284, 291,
    293, 338, 364
  False: 347
Pa$_2$—Poignancy
  True: 24, 158, 299, 305, 317, 341,
    365
  False: 111, 268
Pa$_3$—Naiveté
  True: 314
  False: 93, 109, 117, 124, 313, 316,
    319, 348

Scale 8—Schizophrenia

Sc$_{1A}$—Social Alienation
  True: 16, 21, 24, 35, 52, 121, 157,
    212, 241, 282, 305, 312, 324,
    325, 352, 364
  False: 65, 220, 276, 306, 309
Sc$_{1B}$—Emotional Alienation
  True: 76, 104, 202, 301, 339, 355,
    360, 363
  False: 8, 196, 322
Sc$_{2A}$—Lack of Ego Mastery, Cognitive
  True: 32, 33, 159, 168, 182, 335,
    345, 349, 356
  False: 178
Sc$_{2B}$—Lack of Ego Mastery, Conative
  True: 32, 40, 41, 76, 104, 202, 259,
    301, 335, 339, 356
  False: 8, 196, 322
Sc$_{2C}$—Lack of Ego Mastery, Defective
Inhibition
  True: 22, 97, 156, 194, 238, 266,
    291, 303, 352, 354, 360
  False: None

Sc$_3$—Bizarre Sensory Experiences
  True: 22, 33, 47, 156, 194, 210, 251,
    273, 291, 332, 334, 341, 345,
    350
  False: 103, 119, 187, 192, 281, 330

Scale 9—Hypomania

Ma$_1$—Amorality
  True: 143, 250, 271, 277, 298
  False: 289
Ma$_2$—Psychomotor Acceleration
  True: 13, 97, 100, 134, 181, 228,
    238, 266, 268
  False: 111, 119
Ma$_3$—Imperturbability
  True: 167, 222, 240
  False: 105, 148, 171, 180, 267
Ma$_4$—Ego Inflation
  True: 11, 59, 64, 73, 109, 157, 212,
    232, 233
  False: None

Other Scales

Astvn—Assertiveness (Female)
  True: 3, 28, 37, 45, 52, 54, 63, 101,
    122, 137, 163, 172, 178, 269,
    338, 344, 379, 383, 406, 415,
    432, 436, 458, 462, 474, 476,
    478, 481, 508, 513, 561, 562
  False: 22, 58, 64, 95, 98, 99,158,
    208, 209,254, 276, 320, 326,
    370, 394, 459, 463, 464, 468,
    525, 544, 554, 557
5C—Conservatism
  True: None
  False: 19, 26, 28, 80, 89, 112, 117,
    120, 280
L—Lie Scale
  True: None
  False: 15, 30, 45, 60, 75, 90, 105,
    120, 135, 150, 165, 195, 225,
    255, 285

AMac: Alcoholism
True: 6, 27, 34, 50, 56, 57, 58, 61,
      81, 94, 116, 118, 127, 128,
      140, 156, 186, 215, 224, 235,
      243, 251, 263, 283, 309, 413,
      419, 426, 445, 446, 477, 482,
      483, 488, 500, 507, 529, 562
False: 86, 120, 130, 149, 173, 179,
       278, 294, 320, 335, 357, 378,
       460
Cn: Control
True: 6, 20, 30, 56, 67, 105, 116,
      134, 145, 162, 169, 181, 225,
      236, 238, 285, 296, 319, 337,
      382, 411, 418, 436, 446, 447,
      460, 529, 555,
False: 58, 80, 92, 96, 111, 167, 174,
       220, 242, 249, 250, 291, 313,
       360, 378, 439, 444, 483, 488,
       489, 527, 548
E/Cy: Cynicism (males)
True: 11, 28, 35, 89, 117, 157, 206,
      213, 256, 265, 280, 286, 316,
      319, 365, 454, 56
False: 54, 111, 347
E/Cy: Cynicism (females)
True: 11, 35, 89, 117, 183, 209, 213,
      218, 245, 265, 280, 316, 319,
      454, 465,
False: 54, 111, 115, 306, 347
D-S. Depression, subtle
True: 5, 130, 193
False: 30, 39, 58, 64, 80, 89, 98,
       145, 155, 160, 191, 208, 233,
       241, 248, 263, 296
Ho: Hostility
True: 19, 28, 52, 59, 71, 89, 93,
      110, 117, 124, 136, 148, 157,
      183, 226, 244, 250, 252, 265,
      271, 278, 280, 284, 292, 319,
      348, 368, 383, 386, 394, 406,
      410, 411, 426, 436, 438, 447,
      455, 458, 469, 485, 504, 507,
      520, 531, 551, 558
False: 237, 253, 399

C1: Carelessness

Item Pair	Deviant Response
10 – 405	Same
17 – 65	Different
18 – 63	Different
49 – 113	Same
76 – 107	Same
88 – 526	Same
137 – 216	Same
177 – 220	Different
178 – 342	Same
286 – 312	Different
329 – 425	Same
388 – 480	Different

TR: Test-Retest

Item Pair
8 – 318
13 – 290
15 – 314
16 – 315
20 – 310
21 – 308
22 – 326
23 – 288
24 – 333
32 – 328
33 – 323
35 – 331
37 – 302
38 – 311
305 – 366
317 – 362

OH: Overcontrolled Hostility
True: 78, 91, 229, 319, 338, 373,
      394, 425, 488, 559
False: 1, 30, 81, 90, 102, 109, 129,
       130, 141, 165, 181, 183, 290,
       329, 382, 396, 439, 446, 475,
       501, 534
Pe: Pedophilia
True: 16, 53, 67, 76, 95, 106,
      132, 179, 202, 206, 219, 260,
      332, 390, 458, 490
False: 20, 57, 133, 160, 248, 276,
       435, 556

St: Suspiciousness (St)
  True: 27, 35, 110, 121, 123, 136,
         151, 200, 265, 275, 278, 284,
         291, 293, 348, 364, 384, 448
  False: none
WA: Work Attitude
  True: 13, 16, 32, 35, 40, 41, 59, 84,

109, 112, 170, 244, 250, 259,
272, 301, 312, 331, 335, 343,
389, 395, 404, 406, 435, 487,
507, 526, 549
  False: 3, 9, 88, 164, 207, 257, 318,
         407

Scale Title	Acronym	Source
Alcoholism	AMac	MacAndrew (1965)
Amorality	9AMO	Harris & Lingoes (1955)
Assertiveness	Astvn	Ohlson & Wilson (1974)
Authority Conflict	4AC	Harris & Lingoes (1955)
Authority Conflict	AUT	Wiggins (1966)
Bizarre Sensory Experience	8BSE	Harris & Lingoes (1955)
Body Symptoms	TSC/B	Stein (1968)
Carelessness	CI	Green (1978)
Conservatism	5C	Pepper & Strong (1958)
Control	Cn	Cuadra (1956)
Cynicism	E/Cy	Eichman (1961, 1962)
Denial of Social Anxiety	3DSA	Harris & Lingoes (1955)
Dependency	I-De	Unpublished
Depression	DEP	Wiggins (1966)
Depression	TSC/D	Stein (1968)
Depression-Subtle	D-S	Wiener & Harmon (1946)
Dissociation	I-DS	Unpublished
Dominance	I-Do	Unpublished
Family Problems	FAM	Wiggins (1966)
Family Discord	4FD	Harris & Lingoes (1955)
Feminine Interest	FEM	Wiggins (1966)
Hostility	Ho	Cook & Medley (1954)
Hypomania	HYP	Wiggins (1966)
Imperturbability	9IMP	Harris & Lingoes (1955)
Lack of Ego-Mastery, Cognitive	8Cog	Harris & Lingoes (1955)
Lack of Ego-Mastery, Conative	8Con	Harris & Lingoes (1955)
Lie	L	Dahlstrom et al. (1972)
Manifest Hostility	HOS	Wiggins (1966)
Mean Elevation	ME	Modlin (1947)
Mental Dullness	2MD	Harris & Lingoes (1955)
Naivete	6N	Harris & Lingoes (1955)
Need for Affection	3NA	Harris & Lingoes (1955)
Obsessive-Compulsive	I-OC	Unpublished
Organic Syptoms	ORG	Wiggins (1966)
Overcontrolled Hostility	OH	Megargee et al. (1967)
Pedophilia	Pe	Toobert et al. (1959)
Phobias	PHO	Wiggins (1966)
Poignancy	6P	Harris & Lingoes (1955)

Scale Title	Acronym	Source
Poor Health	HEA	Wiggins (1966)
Poor Morale	MOR	Wiggins (1966)
Psychomotor Acceleration	9PMA	Harris & Lingoes (1955)
Psychomotor Retardation	2PR	Harris & Lingoes (1955)
Psychoticism	PSY	Wiggins (1966)
Religious Fundamentalism	REL	Wiggins (1966)
Resentment	TSC/R	Stein (1968)
Self-Concept	I-SC	Unpublished
Severe Reality Distortions	I-RD	Unpublished
Sex Problems	I-SP	Unpublished
Social Alienation	4SOA	Harris & Lingoes (1955)
Social Alienation	8SOA	Harris & Lingoes (1955)
Social Imperturbability	4SI	Harris & Lingoes (1955)
Social Introversion	TSC/I	Stein (1968)
Social Maladjustment	SOC	Wiggins (1966)
Suspiciousness	TSC/S	Stein (1968)
Suspiciousness	S+	Endicott et al. (1969)
Tension	TSC/T	Stein (1968)
Test-Retest	TR	Buechley & Ball (1952)
Work Attitude	WA	Tydlaska & Mengel (1953)

Appendix II

Demographic Description of the Indiana Sample* (Percents)

	Male	Female	% Total
White	83.7	80.4	82.0
Black	16.3	17.6	17.0
Other	—	2.0	1.0
Total	100.0	100.0	100.0
Married	70.5	47.8	58.9
Never married	18.2	17.4	17.8
Divorced	9.1	26.1	17.8
Widowed	—	6.5	3.3
Separated	2.3	2.2	2.2
Age			
Mean	32.2	36.2	34.2
SD	11.18	13.40	12.06
Range	18–66	18–70	18–70
Educational Level			
Mean	12.5	12.5	12.5
SD	1.75	1.93	1.83
Range	9–16	9–18	9–18

*Race and age are based on $N = 51$ for women and $N = 49$ for men. Marital status and educational level are based on $N = 46$ for women and $N = 44$ for men.

Appendix III

Means and Standard Deviations for the Special Scales Based on the Indiana Sample Data

Means and Standard Deviations
for the Female Sample*
N = 100

Scale	Mean	SD
L	3.82	2.50
TR	1.75	2.02
CI	1.63	1.31
ME	49.01	7.52
ME(K)	56.00	6.35
Qu	1.77	3.46
2SD	7.39	4.69
2PR	6.00	1.74
2PM	3.18	1.26
2MD	2.55	2.62
2B	2.55	2.15
3DSA	3.59	1.82
3NA	5.80	2.29
3LM	2.86	2.79
3SC	3.82	3.03
3IA	3.24	1.31
4FD	2.86	2.38
4AC	4.49	1.88
4SI	6.88	2.75
4SOA	6.51	3.04
4SEA	4.49	2.77
5C	5.25	1.75
6PI	2.37	2.11
6P	2.43	1.64
6N	3.98	2.15

Scale	Mean	SD
8SEA	4.02	3.29
8EA	1.29	1.17
8COG	1.14	1.85
8CON	2.16	2.08
8BSE	2.74	2.85
8DIC	1.88	1.88
9AMO	1.61	1.22
9PMA	5.80	1.90
9IMP	3.02	1.64
9EI	3.53	1.51
AMac	23.31	4.58
OH	14.08	3.50
TSC/I	11.10	5.51
TSC/B	6.76	4.89
TSC/S	12.41	5.00
TSC/D	6.49	5.53
TSC/R	7.59	4.55
TSC/T	11.53	6.17
SOC	11.12	5.80
DEP	7.71	5.99
FEM	19.27	3.50
MOR	8.10	4.98
REL	7.00	2.75
AUT	9.33	3.81
PSY	9.33	4.94
ORG	6.69	5.24
FAM	5.47	3.09
HOS	9.22	4.53
PHO	10.41	3.87
HYP	13.88	3.76
HEA	5.63	3.82
I-SP	2.14	1.46
I-RD	1.73	1.49
I-DS	1.02	1.38
I-OC	3.31	1.68
I-SC	3.78	1.86
I-De	3.86	2.09
I-Do	10.04	2.69
S+	3.20	2.56
D-S	10.78	2.66
Ho	21.00	8.05
Astvn	31.00	4.40
WA	11.35	5.44
E/Cy	5.55	2.78
Cn	26.61	4.46

*Norms for the validity measures Qu, TR, and Cl are based on the total normative subgroups of 57 females and 53 males, prior to elimination of cases due to elevated scores on TR and Cl. ME is the mean of T-scores for Scales 1 through 4 and 6 through 8, K-uncorrected. ME(K) is the same index with K-corrected T-scores.

Means and Standard Deviations
or the Indiana Total Subsample
$N = 51$

Scale	Mean	SD
L	3.93	2.38
TR	1.27	1.91
CI	1.59	1.29
ME	49.02	7.14
ME(K)	57.14	6.24
Qu	1.52	3.23
2SD	6.85	4.25
2PR	5.86	1.87
2PM	2.98	1.15
2MD	2.27	2.29
2B	2.23	1.99
3DSA	3.61	1.91
3NA	5.73	2.33
3LM	2.67	2.42
3SC	3.19	2.79
3IA	3.08	1.28
4FD	2.58	2.06
4AC	4.90	1.85
4SI	7.40	2.61
4SOA	6.24	2.92
4SEA	4.54	2.73
5C	4.96	1.73
6PI	2.27	2.09
6P	2.58	1.60
6N	3.76	2.22
8SOA	3.73	3.18
8EA	1.31	1.13
8COG	1.35	1.85
8CON	2.28	2.09
8BSE	2.49	2.76
8DIC	1.82	1.90
9AMO	1.76	1.20
9PMA	5.82	2.06
9IMP	3.56	1.77
9EI	3.68	1.60
AMac	24.18	4.80
OH	13.69	3.43
TSC/I	9.99	5.59
TSC/B	6.12	4.68
TSC/S	12.33	5.25
TSC/D	6.11	5.28
TSC/R	7.12	4.26
TSC/T	11.03	5.97
SOC	10.51	5.67
DEP	7.48	5.63
FEM	14.66	5.88

Scale	Mean	SD
MOR	7.21	4.98
REL	6.82	2.61
AUT	10.06	4.14
PSY	9.53	5.46
ORG	5.99	4.61
FAM	4.95	2.80
HOS	9.33	4.63
PHO	8.86	4.24
HYP	13.93	3.87
HEA	5.69	3.65
I-SP	2.19	1.51
I-RD	1.81	2.00
I-DS	0.87	1.28
I-OC	3.16	1.68
I-SC	3.50	1.87
I-De	3.90	1.88
I-Do	10.65	2.81
S+	2.97	2.53
D-S	10.47	2.71
Ho	21.11	8.06
WA	11.31	5.19
E/Cy	5.81	2.83
Cn	26.38	4.78

Means and Standard Deviations
for the Indiana Male Subsample
$N = 49$

Scale	Mean	SD
L	4.04	2.27
TR	0.75	1.61
CI	1.54	1.26
ME	49.02	6.79
ME(K)	58.32	5.94
Qu	1.24	2.96
2SD	6.28	3.72
2PR	5.71	2.00
2PM	2.77	0.98
2MD	1.98	1.88
2B	1.90	1.77
3DSA	3.63	2.02
3NA	5.65	2.40
3LM	2.47	1.99
3SC	2.53	2.36
3IA	2.92	1.24
4FD	2.28	1.63
4AC	5.33	1.74
4SI	7.94	2.36
4SOA	5.96	2.78

Scale	Mean	SD
4SEA	4.59	2.72
5C	4.65	1.68
6PI	2.16	2.09
6P	2.73	1.55
6N	3.53	2.29
8SOA	3.43	3.07
8EA	1.33	1.11
8COG	1.57	1.84
8CON	2.41	2.12
8BSE	2.22	2.67
8DIC	1.75	1.94
9AMO	1.92	1.17
9PMA	5.84	2.23
9IMP	4.12	1.73
9EI	3.84	1.69
AMac	25.08	4.89
OH	13.29	3.35
TSC/I	8.84	5.48
TSC/B	5.45	4.41
TSC/S	12.24	5.55
TSC/D	5.71	5.03
TSC/R	6.63	3.93
TSC/T	10.51	5.77
SOC	9.88	5.51
DEP	7.24	5.28
FEM	9.86	3.52
MOR	6.28	4.86
REL	6.63	2.47
AUT	10.82	4.37
PSY	9.73	5.99
ORG	5.26	3.77
FAM	4.41	2.37
HOS	9.45	4.77
PHO	7.24	4.04
HYP	13.98	4.03
HEA	5.75	3.50
Pe	6.92	2.46
I-SP	2.24	1.57
I-RD	1.90	2.43
I-DS	0.71	1.17
I-OC	3.00	1.68
I-SC	3.20	1.85
I-De	3.94	1.65
I-Do	11.29	2.81
S+	2.73	2.51
D-S	10.14	2.75
Ho	21.22	8.16
WA	11.26	4.97
E/Cy	6.08	2.88
Cn	26.14	5.12

Appendix IV

Obvious Subtle Ratings for
the Special Scales

Obvious-Subtle Ratings of Special Scales According to Christian, Burkhart, and Gynther (1978)

		Items			
		Total	Subtle*	S%	O-S Rating
2B	Brooding	10	0	0	3.77
2MD	Mental Dullness	15	0	0	3.55
2PM	Physical Malfunctioning	11	2	18	2.88
2PR	Psychomotor Retardation	15	7	47	2.75
2SD	Subjective Depression	30	3	1	3.52
3DSA	Denial of Social Anxiety	6	4	67	2.10
3IA	Inhibition of Aggression	7	5	71	2.39
3LM	Lassitude-Malaise	15	1	7	3.31
3NA	Need for Affection	12	5	42	2.44
3SC	Somatic Complaints	17	2	18	3.26
4SEA	Self-Alienation	15	1	7	3.48
4SI	Social Imperturbability	12	8	67	2.36
4SOA	Social Alienation	18	2	11	3.44
4AC	Authority Conflict	11	5	45	2.74
4FD	Familial Discord	11	3	27	3.02
6N	Naivete	9	6	67	2.31
6PI	Paranoid Ideation	17	0	0	4.16
6P	Poignancy	9	1	11	3.32
8COG	Lack of Ego Mastery, Cognitive	10	0	0	3.74
8CON	Lack of Ego Mastery, Conative	14	1	7	3.67
8DIC	Lack of Ego Mastery, Defect of Inhibition and Control	11	0	0	3.90
8EA	Emotional Alienation	11	1	9	3.91
8OL	Object Loss	32	1	3	3.67

		Items		
		Total	Subtle*	S%	O-S Rating
8SOA	Social Alienation	21	0	0	3.74
8BSE	Sensory Motor Dissociation	20	0	0	3.65
9AMO	Amorality	6	1	17	2.91
9EI	Ego Inflation	9	2	22	3.09
9IMP	Imperturbability	8	5	63	2.28
9PMA	Psychomotor Acceleration	11	4	36	2.75
AUT	Authority Conflict	20	3	15	2.93
DEP	Depression	33	4	12	3.56
FAM	Family Problems	16	3	19	3.12
FEM	Feminine Interests	30	29	97	1.70
HEA	Poor Health	28	7	25	2.91
HOS	Manifest Hostility	27	3	11	3.29
HYP	Hypomania	25	12	48	2.61
MOR	Poor Morale	23	4	17	3.08
ORG	Organic Symptoms	36	6	17	3.18
PHO	Phobias	27	5	19	3.17
PSY	Psychoticism	45	1	2	3.86
REL	Religious Fundamentalism	12	10	83	1.92
SOC	Social Maladjustment	27	12	44	2.56
TSC/A	Autism	23	4	17	3.22
TSC/B	Body Symptoms	32	2	6	3.27
TSC/D	Depression	28	5	18	3.40
TSC/I	Social Introversion	26	12	46	2.56
TSC/R	Resentment	20	4	20	3.19
TSC/S	Suspicion	25	4	16	2.90
TSC/T	Tension	36	0	0	3.48
I-DS	Dissociation	8	1	13	3.90
I-OC	Obsessive-Compulsive	9	0	0	3.41
I-RD	Severe Distortion of Reality	18	1	6	4.11
I-SC†	Poor Self-Concept (male)	12	0	0	3.55
	(female)	12	0	0	3.52
I-SP	Sex Problems (male)	14	0	0	3.59
	(female)	12	0	0	3.91
I-De	Dependency	9	5	56	2.65
I-Do	Dominance	17	13	76	2.38
AMac	Alcoholism	51	25	49	2.63
Cn	Control	50	26	52	2.63
Ho	Hostility	50	9	18	2.98
Astvn	Assertiveness (Female)	57	35	61	2.43
OH	Overcontrolled Hostility	31	19	61	2.39
Pe	Pedophilia	24	9	38	2.83
S+	Extreme Suspiciousness	18	3	17	3.66
WA	Work a Attitude	37	6	16	3.25
E/Cy	Cynicism (male)	20	4	20	3.42
	(female)	20	4	20	3.46
5C	Conservatism	9	7	78	2.46
D-S	Depression, Subtle	20	14	70	2.21

*Christian, Burkhart, and Gynther (1978) rating of 2.50 or less
†Discrepancy is a function of Item 74.

Appendix V

Special Scales *Not* Recommended for Clinical Use

In addition to the special scales detailed in this book, a number of others have been tested clinically and have been rated as not useful, either with normal groups or with patients. Most have not been subjected to any independent experimental evaluation and none have unequivocal research support. In a few instances, the recommendation does not mean that the scale is inutile per se but only that there are more sensitive scales available in that area.

The Harris and Lingoes scales that should appear in this appendix were identified in Table 3.2 and are not listed again.

References for these scales can be found in Dahlstrom et al. (1975).

A Factor (Welsh)
Admission of Symptoms (Little & Fisher)
Alcoholism (Rosenberg)
Anxiety Index (Welsh)
Autism (Tryon et al.)
Caudality (Williams)
Denial of Symptoms (Little & Fisher)
Dependency (Navran)
Dominance (Gough et al.)
Dominance, revised (Gough et al.)
Ego-Control (Block)

Ego-Resilience (Block)
Ego-Strength (Barron)
Electroshock Prognosis (Feldman)
Extraversion (Giedt & Downing)
Facilitation-Inhibition (Ullman)
Factors I-III (Eichman)
Homosexuality (Panton)
Index of Psychopathology (Sines & Silver)
Internalization Ratio (Welsh)
Low Back Pain (Hanvik)
Manifest Anxiety (Taylor)
Neuroticism (Winne)
Pepper & Strong Scales (except Altruism)
Pharisiac Virtue (Cook & Medley)
Positive Malingering (Cofer et al.)
Prejudice (Gough)
R Factor (Welsh)
Role-Playing (McClelland)
Rosen Scales (Rosen)
Self-Sufficiency (Wolff)
Six Signs (Peterson)
Social Responsibility (Gough)
Social Status (Gough)
Test-Taking Defensiveness (Hanley)
Wiener & Harmon Obvious-Subtle Scales (except Depression-Subtle)

References

Adams, H. B., & Cooper, G. D. (1962). Three measures of ego strength and prognosis for psychotherapy. *Journal of Clinical Psychology, 18,* 490–494.

Adams, H. B., Cooper, G. D., & Carrera, R. N. (1963). The Rorschach and the MMPI: A concurrent validity study. *Journal of Projective Techniques, 27,* 23–34.

Affleck, D. C., & Garfield, S. L. (1960). The prediction of psychosis with the MMPI. *Journal of Clinical Psychology, 16,* 24–26.

American Psychiatric Association (1952). *Diagnostic and statistical manual: Mental disorders,* Washington, DC.

American Psychiatric Association (1987). *Diagnostic and statistical manual of mental disorders.* (rev. 3rd ed.). Washington, DC.

Apfeldorf, M., & Hunley, P. J. (1975). Application of MMPI alcoholism scales to older alcoholics and problem drinkers. *Journal of Studies on Alcohol, 36,* 645–653.

Archer, R. P. (1984). Use of the MMPI with adolescents: A review of salient issues. *Clinical Psychology Review, 4,* 241–251.

Archer, R. P. (1987). *Using the MMPI with adolescents.* Hillsdale, NJ: Lawrence Erlbaum Associates.

Ardell, D. B. (1977). *High level wellness.* Emmaus, PA: Rodale Press.

Ashton, S. G., & Goldberg, L. R. (1973). In response to Jackson's challenge: The comparative validity of personality scales constructed by the external (empirical) strategy & scales developed intuitively by experts, novices, and laymen. *Journal of Research in Personality, 7,* 1–20.

Barefoot, J. C., Dahlstrom, W. G., & Williams, R. B., Jr. (1983). Hostility, CHD incidence, and total mentality: A 25-year follow-up study of 255 physicians. *Psychosomatic Medicine, 45,* 59–63.

Barger, P. M., & Sechrest, L. B. (1961). Convergent and discriminant validity of four Holtzman Inkblot Test variables. *Journal of Psychological Studies, 12,* 227–236.

Barron, F. (1953). An ego-strength scale which predicts response to psychotherapy. *Journal of Consulting Psychology, 17,* 327–333.

Beck, S. J. (1952). Rorschach's Test. III. *Advances in interpretation.* New York: Grune & Stratton.

115

Beck, S. J., Rabin, A. I., Thiesen, W. G., Molish, H. B., & Thetford, W. N. (1950). The normal personality as projected in the Rorschach test. *Journal of Psychology, 30*, 241–298.

Blackburn, R. (1968). Personality in relation to extreme aggression in psychiatric offenders. *British Journal of Psychiatry, 114*, 821–828.

Blackburn, R. (1972). Dimensions of hostility and aggression in abnormal offenders. *Journal of Consulting & Clinical Psychology, 21*, 282–283.

Blanton, R., & Landsman, T. (1952). The re-test reliability of the Group Rorschach and some relationships to the MMPI. *Journal of Consulting Psychology, 16*, 265–267.

Block, J. (1965). *The challenge of response sets.* New York: Appleton-Century-Crofts.

Boerger, A. R. (1975). *The utility of some alternative approaches to MMPI scale construction.* Unpublished doctoral dissertation, Kent State University, Kent, OH.

Bond, J. A. (1986). Inconsistent responding to repeated MMPI items: Is its major cause really carelessness? *Journal of Personality Assessment, 50*, 50–64.

Buechley, R., & Ball, H. (1952). A new test of "validity" for the group MMPI. *Journal of Consulting Psychology, 16*, 299–301.

Burke, H., & Marcus, R. (1977). MacAndrew MMPI Alcoholism Scale: Alcoholism and drug addictiveness. *Journal of Psychology, 96*, 141–148.

Burkhart, B. R., Christian, W. L., & Gynther, M. D. (1978). Item subtlety and faking on the MMPI: a paradoxical relationship. *Journal of Personality Assessment, 42*, 76–80.

Buss, A. H., & Durkee, A. (1957). An inventory for assessing different kinds of hostility. *Journal of Consulting Psychology, 21*, 343–349.

Butcher, J. N., & Tellegen, A. (1978). Common methodological problems in MMPI research. *Journal of Consulting Psychology, 46*, 620–628.

Calvin, J. (1975). *A replicated study of the concurrent validity of the Harris subscales for the MMPI.* Unpublished doctoral dissertation, Kent State University, Kent, OH.

Cernovsky, Z. (1986). Masculinity-femininity scale of the MMPI and intellectual functioning of female addicts. *Journal of Clinical Psychology, 42*, 310–312.

Christian, W. L., Burkhart, B. R., & Gynther, M. D. (1978). Subtle-obvious ratings of MMPI items: New interest in an old concept. *Journal of Clinical Psychology, 46*, 1178–1186.

Clark, J. H. (1948). Some MMPI correlates of color responses in the group Rorschach. *Journal of Consulting Psychology, 12*, 384–386.

Clopton, J. R. (1979a). Development of special MMPI scales. In C. S. Newmark (Ed.), *MMPI clinical and research trends.* New York: Praeger.

Clopton, J. R. (1979b). MMPI and suicide. In C. S. Newmark (Ed.), *MMPI clinical and research trends.* New York: Praeger.

Clopton, J. R., & Neuringer, C. (1979). MMPI cannot say scores: Normative data and degree of profile distortion. *Journal of Personality Assessment, 41*, 511–513.

Colligan, R. C., Osborne, D., Swenson, W. M., & Offord, K. P. (1983). *The MMPI: A contemporary normative study.* New York: Praeger.

Cook, W. W., & Medley, D. M. (1954). Proposed hostility and Pharisaic-virtue scales for the MMPI. *Journal of Applied Psychology, 38*, 414–418.

Costa, P. T., Jr., Zonderman, A. B., McCrae, R. R., & Williams, R. B., Jr. (1985). Content and comprehensiveness in the MMPI: An item factor analysis in a normal adult sample. *Journal of Personality & Social Psychology, 48*, 925–933.

Crumpton, E., Cantor, J. M., & Batiste, C. (1960). A factor analytic study of Barron's Ego-Strength Scale. *Journal of Clinical Psychology, 16*, 283–291.

Cuadra, C. A. (1956). A scale for control in psychological adjustment. In G. S. Welsh & W. G. Dahstrom (Eds.), *Basic readings on the MMPI in psychology and medicine.* Minneapolis: University of Minnesota Press.

Cutter, F. (1957). Rorschach sex responses and overt deviations. *Journal of Clinical Psychology, 13*, 83–86.

Dahlstrom, W. G. (1969). Recurrent issues in the development of the MMPI. In J. N. Butcher

(Ed.), *MMPI: Research developments and clinical applications.* New York: McGraw-Hill.

Dahlstrom, W. G., & Welsh, G. S. (1960). *An MMPI handbook: A guide to use in clinical practice and research.* Minneapolis: University of Minnesota Press.

Dahlstrom, W. G., Welsh, G. S., & Dahlstrom, L. E. (1972). *An MMPI handbook. Vol. I. Clinical interpretation (rev. ed.).* Minneapolis: University of Minnesota Press.

Dahlstrom, W. G., Welsh, G. S., & Dahlstrom, L. E. (1975). *An MMPI handbook. Vol. II. Research applications (rev. ed.).* Minneapolis: University of Minnesota Press.

Dana, R. H. & Bolton, B. (1982). Interrelationships between Rorschach and MMPI scores for female college women. *Psychological Reports, 51,* 1281–1282

deGroot, G. W., & Adamson, J. D. (1973). Responses of psychiatric inpatients to the MacAndrew alcoholism scale. *Quarterly Journal of Studies on Alcohol, 34,* 1133–1139.

Dembroski, T. M., MacDougall, J. M., Williams, R. B., Jr., & Haney, T. (1985). Components of Type A, hostility and anger-in: Relationship to angiographic findings. *Psychosomatic Medicine, 47,* 219–233.

deMendonca, M., Elliott, L., Goldstein, M., McNeill, J., Rodriguez, R., & Zelkind, I. (1984). An MMPI-based behavior descriptor/personality trait list. *Journal of Personality Assessment, 48,* 483–485.

Duckworth, J. C., & Anderson, W. P. (1986). *MMPI interpretation manual for counselors and clinicians (3rd ed.).* Muncie, IN: Accelerated Development.

Edwards, A. L. (1959). *Edwards Personal Preference Schedule.* New York: The Psychological Corp.

Eichman, W. J. (1961). Replicated factors on the MMPI with female NP patients. *Journal of Consulting Psychology, 25,* 55–60.

Eichman, W. J. (1962). Factored scales for the MMPI: A clinical and statistical manual. *Journal of Clinical Psychology, 18,* 363–395.

Endicott, N. A., Jortner, A. S., & Abramoff, E. (1969). Objective measures of suspiciousness. *Journal of Abnormal Psychology, 74,* 26–32.

Exner, J. E. (1978). *The Rorschach: A comprehensive system (Vol. 2,).* New York: Wiley.

Exner, J. E. (1986). *The Rorschach: A comprehensive system (Vol. 1, 2nd ed.).* New York: Wiley.

Farberow, N. L., & Devries, A. G. (1967). An item differentiation analysis of suicidal neuropsychiatric hospital patients. *Psychological Reports, 20,* 607–617.

Faschingbauer, T. R. (1979). The future of the MMPI. In C. S. Newmark (Ed.), *MMPI clinical and research trends.* New York: Praeger.

Fisher, G. (1970). Discriminating violence emanating from over-controlled versus undercontrolled aggressivity. *British Journal of Social & Clinical Psychology, 18,* 140–141.

Foerstner, S. B. (1986). *The factor structure and factor stability of selected Minnesota Multiphasic Personality Inventory (MMPI) subscales: Harris and Lingoes subscales, Wiggins content scales, Weiner subscales, and Serkownek subscales.* Unpublished doctoral dissertation, University of Akron, Akron, OH.

Forsyth, R. P., Jr. (1959). The influence of color, shading and Welsh anxiety level on Elizer Rorschach Content Test analysis of anxiety and hostility. *Journal of Projective Techniques & Personality Assessment, 23,* 207–213.

Fredericksen, S. J. (1975). *A comparison of selected personality and history variables in highly violent, mildly violent and nonviolent female offenders.* Unpublished doctoral dissertation, University of Minnesota, Minneapolis, MN.

Gebhard, P. H., Gagnon, J. H., Pomeroy, W. B., & Christenson, C. V. (1965). *Sex offenders.* New York: Harper & Row.

Gilberstadt, H., & Duker, J. (1965). *A handbook for clinical and actuarial MMPI interpretation.* Philadelphia: Saunders.

Goldberg, L. R. (1965). Diagnosticians v. diagnostic signs: The diagnosis of psychosis vs. neurosis from the MMPI. *Psychological Monographs, 79,* 9 (Whole No. 602).

Goldfried, M. R., Stricker, G., & Weiner, I. B. (1971). *Rorschach handbook of clinical and research application.* Englewood Cliffs, NJ: Prentice-Hall.

Goodstein, L. D., & Goldberger, L. (1955). Manifest anxiety and Rorschach performance in a chronic patient population. *Journal of Consulting Psychology, 19,* 339–344.

Gottesman, I. I., Hanson, D. R., Kroeker, T. A., & Briggs, P. E. (1987). New MMPI normative data and power-transformed *T*-score tables for the Hathaway-Monachesi Minnesota cohort of 14,019 15-year-olds and 3,674 18-year-olds. In Archer, R. P. *Using the MMPI with adolescents.* Hillsdale, NJ: Lawrence Erlbaum Associates.

Gough, H. G. (1950). The F minus K dissimulation index for the Minnesota Multiphasic Personality Inventory. *Journal of Consulting Psychology, 14,* 408–413.

Graham, J. R. (1977). *The MMPI: A practical guide.* New York: Oxford University Press.

Graham, J. R. (1978). Review of Minnesota Multiphasic Personality Inventory special scales. In P. McReynolds (Ed.), *Advances in psychological assessment.* San Francisco: Jossey-Bass.

Graham, J. R. (1987). *The MMPI: A practical guide,* (2nd ed.). New York: Oxford University Press.

Gravitz, M. A. (1970). Validity implications of normal adult MMPI "L" Scale endorsement. *Journal of Clinical Psychology, 26,* 497–499.

Grayson, H. M. (1951). *A psychological admissions testing program and manual.* Los Angeles: Veterans Administration Center, Neuropsychiatric Hospital.

Greenberg, J. S. (1985). Health and wellness: A conceptual differentiation. *Journal of School Health, 55,* 403–406.

Greene, R. L. (1978). An empirically derived MMPI Carelessness Scale. *Journal of Clinical Psychology, 34,* 407–410.

Greene, R. L. (1979). Response consistency on the MMPI: The TR Index. *Journal of Personality Assessment, 43,* 69–71.

Greene, R. L. (1980). *The MMPI: An interpretive manual.* New York: Grune & Stratton.

Grosz, H. J., & Levitt, E. E. (1959). The effects of hypnotically induced anxiety on the Manifest Anxiety Scale and the Barron Ego-Strength Scale. *Journal of Abnormal & Social Psychology, 59,* 281–283.

Gynther, M. D., Burkhart, B. R., & Hovanitz, C. (1979). Do face-valid items have more predictive validity than subtle items? The case of the MMPI *Pd* Scale. *Journal of Consulting & Clinical Psychology, 47,* 295–300.

Harris, R. E., & Lingoes, J. C. (1955). *Subscales for the MMPI: An aid to profile interpretation (mimeographed).* San Francisco, CA: Department of Psychiatry, University of California. (rev. ed. 1968).

Hathaway, S. R. (1947). A coding system for MMPI profiles. *Journal of Consulting Psychology, 11,* 334–337.

Hathaway, S. R., & McKinley, J. C. (1951). *Minnesota Multiphasic Personality Inventory Manual (revised).* New York: The Psychological Corp.

Hathaway, S. R., & McKinley, J. C. (1983). *Minnesota Multiphasic Personality Inventory Manual for Administration and Scoring.* Minneapolis: University of Minnesota Press.

Hathaway, S. R., & Monachesi, E. D. (1963). *Adolescent personality and behavior: MMPI patterns of normal, delinquent, dropout and other outcomes.* Minneapolis, MN: University of Minnesota Press.

Hawkinson, J. R. (1961). A study of the construct validity of Barron's Ego-Strength Scale with a state mental hospital population. *Dissertation Abstracts, 22,* 4031.

Haven, H. J. (1972). *Descriptive and developmental characteristics of chronically overcontrolled hostile prisoners.* Unpublished doctoral dissertation, Florida State University, Tallahassee, FL.

Haymond, P. J. (1981). *A new look at an old team: A correlational study of the Rorschach and MMPI with adolescent female delinquents.* Unpublished doctoral dissertation, Indiana

University, Bloomington, IN.

Heist, P., & Yonge, G. (1968). *Manual for the Omnibus Personality Inventory.* New York: The Psychological Corp.

Herron, W. G., Guido, S. M., & Kantor, R. C. (1965). Relationships among ego strength measures. *Journal of Psychological Studies, 13,* 173–203.

Hoffman, H., Loper, R. G., & Kammeier, M. L. (1974). Identifying future alcoholics with MMPI alcohol scales. *Quarterly Journal of Studies on Alcohol, 35,* 490–498.

Hollandsworth, J. G. (1977). Differentiating assertion and aggression: Some behavioral guidelines. *Behavior Therapy, 8,* 347–352.

Hollandsworth, J. G., & Wall, K. E. (1977). Sex differences in assertive behavior: an empirical investigation. *Journal of Counseling Psychology, 24,* 217–222.

Huber, N., & Danahy, S. (1975). Use of the MMPI in predicting completion and evaluating changes in a long-term alcoholism treatment program. *Journal of Studies on Alcohol, 36,* 1230–1237.

Huff, F. W. (1965). Use of actuarial description of abnormal personality in a mental hospital. *Psychological Reports, 17,* 224.

Jackson, D. N. (1975). The relative validity of scales prepared by naive item writers and those based on empirical methods of personality scale construction. *Educational & Psychological Measurement, 35,* 361–370.

Jarneke, R. W., & Chambers, E. D. (1977). MMPI content scales: Dimensional structure, construct validity, and interpretive norms in a psychiatric population. *Journal of Consulting & Clinical Psychology, 45,* 1126–1131.

Johnson, J. S., Null, C., Butcher, J. N., & Johnson, K. N. (1984). Replicated item level factor analysis of the full MMPI. *Journal of Personality & Social Psychology, 47,* 105–114.

Jurjevich, R. M. (1963). Relationships among the MMPI and HGI hostility scales. *Journal of General Psychology, 69,* 131–133.

Kammeier, M. L., Hoffman, H., & Loper, R. G. (1973). Personality characteristics of alcoholics as college freshmen and at time of treatment. *Quarterly Journal of Studies on Alcohol, 34,* 390–399.

King-Ellison Good, P. E. (1957). A psychological study of the effects of regressive electroshock treatment. *Dissertation Abstracts, 17,* 2064–2065.

Kleinmuntz, B. (1960). An extension of the construct validity of the ego–strength scale. *Journal of Consulting Psychology, 24,* 463–464.

Klerman, G. L. (1982). Practical issues in the treatment of depression and mania. In E. S. Paykel (Ed.), *Handbook of affective disorders.* New York: Churchill Livingstone.

Klopfer, B., Kirkner, F. J., Wisham, W., & Baker, G. (1954). Rorschach Prognostic Rating Scale. In B. Klopfer, M. D. Ainsworth, W. G. Klopfer, & R. R. Holt (Eds.), *Developments in the Rorschach Technique (Vol. 1).* Yonkers-on-Hudson, NY: World Book Co.

Klopfer, B., & Spiegelman, M. (1956). Differential diagnosis. In B. Klopfer (Ed.), *Developments in the Rorschach technique: Fields of application (Vol. 2).* Yonkers-on-Hudson, NY: World Book Co.

Kobasa, S. C. (1979). Stressful life events, personality, and health: An inquiry into hardiness. *Journal of Personality & Social Psychology, 37,* 1–11.

Kobasa, S. C. (1982). The hardy personality: Toward a social psychology of stress and health. In G. S. Sanders & J. Suls (Eds.), *Social psychology of health and illness.* Hillsdale, NJ: Lawrence Erlbaum Associates.

Koss, M. P, Butcher, J. N., & Hoffman, N. G. (1976). The MMPI critical items: How well do they work? *Journal of Consulting & Clinical Psychology, 44,* 921–928.

Kranitz, L. (1972). Alcoholics, heroin addicts, and nonaddicts: Comparisons on the MacAndrew alcoholism scale of the MMPI. *Quarterly Journal of Studies on Alcohol, 33,* 908–909.

Lachar, D., & Alexander, P. S. (1978). Veridicality of self-report: replicated correlates of the

Wiggins MMPI Content Scales. *Journal of Consulting & Clinical Psychology, 46,* 1349-1356.

Lachar, D., Berman, W., Grisell, J. L., & Schooff, K. (1976). The MacAndrew Alcoholism Scale as a general measure of substance abuse. *Journal of Studies on Alcohol, 37,* 1609-1615.

Lachar, D., Klinge, V., & Grisell, J. L. (1976). Relative accuracy of automated MMPI narratives generated from adult norm and adolescent norm profiles. *Journal of Consulting & Clinical Psychology, 44,* 20-24.

Lachar, D., Lewis, R., & Kupke, T. (1979). MMPI in differentiation of temporal lobe and nontemporal lobe epilepsy: Investigation of three levels of test performance. *Journal of Consulting & Clinical Psychology, 47,* 186-188.

Lane, P. J., & Kling, J. S. (1979). Construct validity of the Overcontrolled Hostility Scale of the MMPI. *Journal of Consulting & Clinical Psychology, 47,* 781-782.

Leavitt, F. & Garron, D. C. (1982). Rorschach and Pain characteristics of patients with low back pain and "conversion VMMPI profiles." *Journal of Personality Assessment, 46,* 18-25.

Lebovits, B. Z., & Ostfeld, A. M. (1967). Personality, defensiveness and educational achievement. *Journal of Personality & Social Psychology, 6,* 381-390.

Lebovits, B. Z., Visotsky, H. M., & Ostfeld, A. M. (1960). LSD and JB 318: A comparison of two hallucinogens. *Archives of General Psychiatry, 2,* 390-407.

Lester, D., Perdue, W. C., & Brookhart, D. (1974). Murder and the control of aggression. *Psychological Reports, 34,* 706.

Levine, D., & Cohen, J. (1962). Symptoms and ego strength measures as predictors of the outcome of hospitalization in functional psychoses. *Journal of Consulting Psychology, 26,* 246-250.

Levitt, E. E. (1980a). *Primer on the Rorschach technique: a method of administration, scoring and interpretation.* Springfield, IL: Thomas.

Levitt, E. E. (1980b). *The psychology of anxiety. (2nd ed.)* Hillsdale, NJ: Lawrence Erlbaum Associates.

Levitt, E. E., & Duckworth, J. C. (1984). Minnesota Multiphasic Personality Inventory. In D. J. Keyser & R. C. Sweetland (Eds.), *Test critiques (Vol. 1).* Kansas City, MO: Test Corporation of America.

Levitt, E. E., Lubin, B., & Brooks, J. M. (1983). *Depression: concepts, controversies and some new facts (2nd ed.).* Hillsdale, NJ: Lawrence Erlbaum Associates.

Lingoes, J. C. (1960). MMPI factors of the Harris and the Wiener Subscales. *Journal of Consulting Psychology, 24,* 74-83.

Loper, R. G., Kammeier, M. L., & Hoffmann, H. (1973). MMPI characteristics of college freshman males who later became alcoholics. *Journal of Abnormal Psychology, 82,* 159-162.

Lothstein, L. M., & Jones, P. (1978). Discriminating violent individuals by means of various psychological tests. *Journal of Personality Assessment, 42,* 237-243.

Lubin, B., Larsen, R. M., & Matarazzo, J. D. (1983). Psychological test usage in the United States: 1935-1982. *American Psychologist, 39,* 451-454.

MacAndrew, C. (1965). The differentiation of male alcoholic outpatients from nonalcoholic psychiatric outpatients by means of the MMPI. *Quarterly Journal of Studies on Alcohol, 26,* 238-246.

Mallory, C. H., & Walker, C. E. (1972). MMPI O–H scale responses of assaultive and nonassaultive prisoners and associated life history variables. *Educational & Psychological Measurement, 32,* 1125-1128.

Marks, P., & Seeman, W. (1963). *The actuarial description of abnormal personality.* Baltimore: Williams & Wilkins.

Marks, P., Seeman, W., & Haller, D. L. (1974). *The actuarial use of the MMPI with adolescents and adults.* Baltimore: Williams & Wilkins.

McCreary, C. P. (1975). Personality differences among child molesters. *Journal of Personality Assessment, 39,* 591–593.

McGee, S. (1954). Measurement of hostility: a pilot study. *Journal of Clinical Psychology, 10,* 280–282.

Meehl, P. E., & Dahlstrom, W. G. (1960). Objective configural rules for discriminating psychotic from neurotic MMPI profiles. *Journal of Consulting Psychology, 24,* 375–387.

Megargee, E. I. (1966). Undercontrolled and overcontrolled personality types in extreme antisocial aggression. *Psychological Monographs, 80,* 3 (Whole No. 611).

Megargee, E. I. (1969). Conscientious objector's scores on the MMPI O-H scale. *Proceedings of the 77th Annual Convention of the American Psychological Association, 4,* 507–508.

Megargee, E. I., Cook, P. E. & Mendelsohn, G. A. (1967). The development and validation of an MMPI scale of assaultiveness in overcontrolled individuals. *Journal of Abnormal Psychology, 72,* 519–528.

Megargee, E. I., & Mendelsohn, G. A. (1962). A cross-validation of twelve MMPI indexes of hostility and control. *Journal of Abnormal & Social Psychology, 65,* 431–438.

Mezzich, J. E., Damarin, F. L., & Erickson, J. R. (1974). Comparative validity strategies and indices for differential diagnosis of depressive states from other psychiatric conditions using the MMPI. *Journal of Consulting & Clinical Psychology, 42,* 691–698.

Modlin, H. C. (1947). A study of the Minnesota Multiphasic Personality Inventory in clinical practice with notes on the Cornell Index. *American Journal of Psychiatry, 103,* 758–769.

Moos, R. H., & Solomon, G. F. (1964). Minnesota Multiphasic Personality Inventory response pattern in patients with rheumatoid arthritis. *Journal of Psychosomatic Research, 8,* 17–28.

Moreland, K. L., & Dahlstrom, W. G. (1983). Professional training with and use of the MMPI. *Professional Psychology, 14,* 218–223.

Navran, L. (1954). A rationally derived MMPI scale to measure dependence. *Journal of Consulting Psychology, 18,* 192.

Norman, W. T. (1972). Psychometric considerations for a revision of the MMPI. In J. N. Butcher (Ed.), *Objective personality assessment.* New York: Academic Press.

Ohlson, E. L., & Wilson, M. (1974). Differentiating female homosexuals from female heterosexuals by use of the MMPI. *Journal of Sex Research, 10,* 308–315.

Palmer, W. G. (1970). *Actuarial interpretation of the MMPI: a replication and extension.* Unpublished doctoral dissertation, University of Alabama, Tuscaloosa, AL.

Pancoast, D. L., Archer, R. P., & Gordon, R. A. (1988). The MMPI and clinical diagnosis: A comparison of classification system outcomes with discharge diagnoses. *Journal of Personality Assessment, 52,* 81–90.

Panton, J. H. (1959). The response of prison inmates to MMPI subscales. *Journal of Social Therapy, 5,* 233–237.

Payne, F. D., & Wiggins, J. S. (1972). MMPI profile types and the self-report of psychiatric patients. *Journal of Abnormal Psychology, 29,* 1–8.

Pepper, L. J., & Strong, P. N. (1958). *Judgmental subscales for the Mf scale of the MMPI.* Unpublished manuscript.

Peterson, D. R. (1954). Predicting hospitalization of psychiatric outpatients. *Journal of Abnormal & Social Psychology, 49,* 260–265.

Pokorny, A. D. (1968). Myths about suicide. In H. L. P. Resnik (Ed.), *Suicidal behavior: diagnosis and management.* Boston, Little Brown.

Quay, H. (1955). The performance of hospitalized psychiatric patients on the ego-strength scale of the MMPI. *Journal of Clinical Psychology, 11,* 403–405.

Rawlings, M. L. (1973). Self control and interpersonal violence: A study of Scottish adolescent male severe offenders. *Criminology, 11,* 23–48.

Reading, E. A. (1978). *The Rorschach and the MMPI: A construct validity study.* Unpublished master's thesis, University of South Florida, Tampa, FL.

Rhodes, R. J. (1969). The MacAndrew alcoholism scale: A replication. *Journal of Clinical Psychology, 25,* 489–491.

Rice, D. G. (1968). Rorschach responses and aggressive characteristics of MMPI *F* 16 scorers. *Journal of Projective Techniques & Personality Assessment, 32,* 253–261.

Rice, D. G., Slembach, R. A., & Pann, N. E. (1969). Comparative diagnostic judgment from the Rorschach and the MMPI. *Journal of Projective Techniques & Personality Assessment, 32,* 253–261.

Rich, C. C., & Davis, H. G. (1969). Concurrent validity of MMPI alcoholism scales. *Journal of Clinical Psychology, 25,* 425–426.

Rosen, A. (1962). Development of the MMPI scales based on a reference group of psychiatric patients. *Psychological Monographs, 76,* 8 (Whole No. 527).

Rosen, A. (1963). Diagnostic differentiation as a construct validity indicator for the MMPI ego-strength scale. *Journal of General Psychology, 69,* 293–297.

Rosen, E. (1952). MMPI and Rorschach correlates of the Rorschach white space response. *Journal of Clinical Psychology, 8,* 283–288.

Schuerger, J. M., Foerstner, S. B., Serkownek, K., & Ritz, G. (1987). History and validities of the Serkownek subscales for MMPI Scales 5 and 0. *Psychological Reports, 61,* 227–235.

Shaw, M. C., & Grubb, J., (1958). Hostility and able high school underachievers. *Journal of Counseling Psychology, 5,* 263–266.

Shekelle, R. B., Gale, M., Ostfeld, A. M., & Paul, O. (1983). Hostility, risk of coronary heart disease, and mortality. *Psychosomatic Medicine, 45,* 109–114.

Shipman, W. G. (1965). The validity of MMPI hostility scales. *Journal of Clinical Psychology, 21,* 186–190.

Sines, L. K., & Silver, R. J. (1963). An index of psychopathology (IP) derived from clinician's judgments of MMPI profiles. *Journal of Clinical Psychology, 19,* 324–326.

Sinnett, E. R. (1962). The relationship between the Ego–Strength Scale and rated in-hospital improvement. *Journal of Clinical Psychology, 18,* 46–47.

Smith, W. H., & Coyle, F. A., Jr. (1969). MMPI and Rorschach form level scores in a student population. *Journal of Psychology, 73,* 3–7.

Smith, T. W., & Frohm, K. D. (1985). What's so unhealthy about hostility? construct validity and psychosocial correlates of the Cook and Medley Ho Scale. *Health Psychology, 4,* 503–520.

Snow, D. L., & Held, M. L. (1973). Relation between locus of control and the MMPI with obese female adolescents. *Journal of Clinical Psychology, 29,* 24–25.

Spielberger, C. D., Jacobs, G. A., Russell, S., & Crane, R. S. (1983). Assessment of anger: The State-Trait Anger Scale. In J. N. Butcher & C. D. Spielberger (Eds.), *Advances in personality assessment (Vol. 2).* Hillsdale, NJ: Lawrence Erlbaum Associates.

Stein, K. B. (1968). The TSC Scales: The outcome of a cluster analysis of the 550 MMPI items. In P. McReynolds (Ed.): *Advances in psychological assessment (Vol. 1).* Palo Alto, CA: Science & Behavior Books.

Sundberg, N. D. (1961). The practice of psychological testing in clinical services in the United States. *American Psychologist, 16,* 79–83.

Sutker, P. B., & Allain, A. N. (1979). MMPI Studies of extreme criminal violence in incarcerated women and men. In C. S. Newmark (Ed.), *MMPI clinical and research trends.* New York: Praeger.

Svanum, S., Levitt, E. E., & McAdoo, W. G. (1982). Differentiating male and female alcoholics from psychiatric outpatients: the MacAndrew and Rosenberg alcoholism scales. *Journal of Personality Assessment, 46,* 81–84.

Taft, R. (1957). The validity of the Barron Ego-Strength Scale and the Welsh Anxiety Index. *Journal of Consulting Psychology, 21,* 247–249.

Tamkin, A. S. (1957). An evaluation of the construct validity of Barron's ego–strength scale.

Journal of Clinical Psychology, 13, 156–158.

Tamkin, A. S., & Klett, C. J. (1957). Barron's Ego-Strength Scale: A replication of an evaluation of its construct validity. *Journal of Consulting Psychology, 21,* 412.

Taulbee, E. S. (1961). The relationship between Rorschach flexor and extensor M. responses and the MMPI and psychotherapy. *Journal of Projective Techniques, 25,* 477–479.

Taylor, J. A. (1953). A personality scale of manifest anxiety. *Journal of Abnormal & Social Psychology, 48,* 285–290.

Taylor, J. B., Ptacek, M., Carithers, M., Griffin, G., & Coyne, L. (1972). Rating scales as measures of clinical judgment: III. Judgments of the self on personality inventory scales and direct ratings. *Educational and Psychological Measurement, 32,* 543–557.

Tesseneer, R., & Tydlaska, M. (1956). A cross-validation of a work attitude scale from the MMPI. *Journal of Educational Psychology, 47,* 1–7.

Thompson, G. M. (1948). MMPI correlates of certain movement responses in the group Rorschach of two college samples. *Journal of Consulting Psychology, 12,* 379–383.

Toobert, S., Bartelme, K. F., & Jones, E. S. (1959). Some factors related to pedophilia. *International Journal of Social Psychiatry, 4,* 272–279.

Tryon, R. C. (1966). Unrestricted cluster and factor analysis with application to the MMPI and Holzinger-Harman problems. *Multivariate Behavioral Research, 1,* 229–244.

Tydlaska, M., & Mengel, R. (1953). A scale for measuring work attitudes for the MMPI. *Journal of Applied Psychology, 37,* 474–477.

Uecker, A. E. (1970). Differentiating male alcoholics from other psychiatric inpatients: validity of the MacAndrew scale. *Quarterly Journal of Studies on Alcohol, 31,* 379–383.

Vanderbeck, D. J., (1973). A construct validity study of the O-H Scale of the MMPI, using a social learning approach to the catharsis effect. *FCI Research Reports, 5,* 1–18.

Van Evra, J. P., & Rosenburg, B. G. (1963). Ego strength and ego disjunction in primary and secondary psychopaths. *Journal of Clinical Psychology, 19,* 61–63.

Vega, A. (1971). Cross-validation of four MMPI scales for alcoholism. *Quarterly Journal of Studies on Alcohol, 32,* 791–797.

Wade, T. C., & Baker, T. B. (1977). Opinions and use of psychological tests: A survey of clinical psychologists. *American Psychologist, 32,* 874–882.

Ward, L. C., & Ward, J. W. (1980). MMPI readability reconsidered. *Journal of Personality Assessment, 44,* 387–389.

Welsh, G. S. (1952). An anxiety index and an internationalization ratio for the MMPI. *Journal of Consulting Psychology, 16,* 65–72.

Welsh, G. S. (1956). Factor dimensions A and R. In G. S. Welsh, & W. G. Dahlstrom (Eds.), *Basic readings on the MMPI in psychology and medicine.* Minneapolis: University of Minnesota Press.

Welsh, G. S., & Dahlstrom, W. G. (1956). *Basic readings on the MMPI in psychology and medicine.* Minneapolis: University of Minnesota Press.

Whisler, R. H., & Cantor, J. M. (1966). The MacAndrew alcoholism scale: A cross-validation in a domiciliary setting. *Journal of Clinical Psychology, 22,* 311–312.

White, W. C. (1970). *Selective modeling in youthful offenders with high and low O-H personality types.* Unpublished doctoral dissertation, Florida State University, Tallahassee, FL.

White, W. C. (1975). Validity of the Overcontrolled Hostility (O-H) Scale: A brief report. *Journal of Personality Assessment, 39,* 587–590.

White, W. C., McAdoo, W. G., & Megargee, E. I. (1973). Personality factors associated with over and undercontrolled offenders. *Journal of Personality Assessment, 37,* 473–478.

Wiener, D. N. (1948). Subtle and obvious keys for the MMPI. *Journal of Consulting Psychology, 12,* 164–170.

Wiener, D. N. (1956). Subtle and obvious keys for the MMPI. In G. S. Welsh & W. G. Dahlstrom (Eds.), *Basic readings on the MMPI in psychology and medicine.* Minneapolis:

University of Minnesota Press.

Wiener, D. N., & Harmon, L. R. (1946). *Subtle and obvious keys for the MMPI: Their development*. Minneapolis: VA Advisement Bulletin No. 16.

Wiggins, J. S. (1966). Substantive dimensions of self-report in the MMPI item pool. *Psychological Monographs, 80,* 22 (Whole No. 630).

Wiggins, J. S., Goldberg, L. R., & Applebaum, M. (1971). MMPI content scales: interpretive norms and correlations with other scales. *Journal of Consulting & Clinical Psychology, 37,* 403–410.

Williams, H. L., & Lawrence, J. F. (1954). Comparison of Rorschach and MMPI by means of factor analysis. *Journal of Consulting Psychology, 18,* 193–197.

Williams, R. B., Jr., Haney, T. L., Lee, K. L., Kong, Y., Blumenthal, J. A., & Whalen, R., E. (1980). Type A behavior, hostility and coronary atherosclerosis. *Psychosomatic Medicine, 42,* 539–549.

Winter, W. D., & Stortroen, M. (1963). A comparison of several MMPI indices to differentiate psychotics from normals. *Journal of Clinical Psychology, 19,* 220–223.

Winters, K. C., Weintraub, S., & Neale, J. M. (1981). Validity of MMPI codetypes in identifying DSM-III schizophrenics, unipolars, and bipolars. *Journal of Consulting & Clinical Psychology, 49,* 486–487.

Woodward, W. A., Robinowitz, R., & Penk, W. E. (1980). *Predicting substance abusers' return to treatment from first admission personality scales*. Paper presented at the meeting of the Society for Personality Assessment, Tampa, FL, March.

Wrobel, T. A., & Lachar, D. L. (1982). Validity of the Wiener subtle and obvious scales for the MMPI: another example of the importance of inventory-item content. *Journal of Consulting & Clinical Psychology, 50,* 469–470.

Zimet, C. N., & Brackbill, G. A. (1956). The role of anxiety in psychodiagnosis. *Journal of Clinical Psychology, 12,* 173–177.

Zuckerman, M. (1979). *Sensation seeking: Beyond the optimal level of arousal*. Hillsdale, NJ: Lawrence Erlbaum Associates.

Author Index

Subject Index

Special scales
  and adolescents, 11–13
  neglect of, 6–8
Subjective Depression Scale (2SD) (D1), 24, 60, 61
Suspicion Scale (TSC/S), 43, 64, 65, 70, 72, 93
Symptoms, psychological, *see* Assessment of psychopathology, *see also* Conflict Tension Scale (TSC/T), 43, 59, 89, 93

T

Test-Retest Scale (TR), *see* Measures of validity
Traits, personality, *see* Personality patterns

W

Work Attitude Scale, *see* Prognosis